Melt The Me Middle:

A Beginner's Guide For Women To The Intermittent Fasting & Essential Oils Lifestyle

Jill Lebofsky

Melt The Midlife Middle
Copyright © 2019 by Jill Lebofsky. All rights reserved.

Contents

My Intermittent Fasting Journey

This book isn't meant to be anthology of all things Intermittent Fasting. It is meant to be a beginner's guide for the midlife woman to adapt easily to an Intermittent Fasting lifestyle and become a fat burning machine! There are other books out there that dig deeper into the how and why behind Intermittent Fasting. I have included a list of some of my favorites in the *Resources* chapter, and I strongly encourage you to read them. Those books cover the significant amount of research and science to date in support of Intermittent Fasting (IF), and they address the physiological reasons behind why IF is so effective. They also describe multiple strategies for Intermittent Fasting. This book will focus solely on one method of Intermittent Fasting, the 16/8 method.

I feel strongly that understanding WHY intermittent fasting works is vital to your success. The first half of this book will focus on the basic science behind Intermittent Fasting, why it is the perfect method for sustainable weight loss for the midlife woman, what essential oils are and which ones are most beneficial to supporting weight management efforts. This second half will focus on the simple – but entirely effective – 16/8 method. What exactly is the 16/8 method? Simply put, you do all your eating during an 8-hour window of time, and then for 16 hours you eat nothing. (The best part is that you'll be sleeping for 8 of those 16 hours which is half your fasting time!) Why would anyone eat this way, you ask? The benefits to intermittent fasting can be life changing, from clearer thinking to healthy, long-term weight loss.

I focus on three primary elements when I teach the 16/8 method:

1. What you do during the fast (the part of the day when you are NOT eating)

2. What you do during the eating window (the part of the day when you ARE eating)

3. Learning to listen to your body and gauge your hunger/satisfaction level.

By the end of this book, you will be fully equipped with the knowledge of how and why Intermittent Fasting works, with the tools to successfully incorporate the 16/8 method into your life and for getting rid of the midlife middle for good.

This book is designed as a practical Intermittent Fasting beginner's guide for a specific group near and dear to my heart: the midlife woman. Most of the existing literature on Intermittent Fasting is written for the general population, and doesn't attempt to differentiate between the sometimes opposing needs of the two sexes. The truth is, men and women ARE different. Our very motivations for losing weight are often different. HOW we lose weight is different. Right? Have you ever worked your butt off, dieting and exercising, only to see the scale move a pound or two . . . and then your husband announces he's going on a diet, skips lunch, goes to the bathroom and loses five pounds? That is so annoying!! In addition, we midlife women experience an inevitable life change that causes us to lose weight differently than our younger counterparts.

Women over 40 go through the unique experience of menopause. In my first book, "No Sweat It's Just Menopause: Eating, Exercise & Essential Oils For A Healthy Change," I cover how this normal, biological transition typically begins when a woman reaches her early to mid-40's, and can last between 6 to 10 years. Available at **bit.ly/naturalmenopausebook**, it nicely complements this book. Whether you're in perimenopause (you've started to skip periods and notice physical and emotional changes) or post-menopause (defined as more than 12 months since your last period), depleted estrogen, hormonal imbalance, and stress due to life changes all contribute to stubborn fat forming around the midsection, setting up camp, and not budging despite your best efforts.

I just described myself: After maintaining my ideal weight for 12 years, I hit my mid-40's, and my periods became sporadic. I began to experience hot flashes and mood swings. The number on my scale slowly climbed until I found myself 20 pounds overweight, wondering if I would keep getting bigger and bigger. I hadn't really changed my eating or exercise habits, but the habits I always depended on to keep me trim and fit no longer worked. For many years, my middle aged Pilates and health coaching clients swore to me that they were doing everything right – eating healthy, watching their portions, exercising regularly – and yet they weren't losing weight. I hate to admit it, but in hindsight I probably doubted their commitment and figured they weren't being completely honest with themselves or with me about their efforts – because if they were, they'd shed the pounds. Right? Boy, was I wrong about that!

When I first learned about Intermittent Fasting, around my 48th birthday, I began researching its history, methods, and effects like a woman on a mission. I'd been teaching healthy eating strategies to clients for a long time, starting as a Weight Watchers leader for many years, then as a women's health coach, teaching my own healthy eating methods with a plant-based focus. When I heard the words "Intermittent Fasting," I nearly dismissed it as unsafe, unhealthy weight loss. For years, I had preached to my clients the line I had been taught: "If you don't eat often enough, your body will believe it is going to starve and it starts holding onto the fat." Now I know that is simply not true.

As I continued to learn more about Intermittent Fasting, I discovered how misguided my thinking had been. I gained a better understanding of what Intermittent Fasting is, and how in addition to being a completely safe and viable way to lose weight, it has other health benefits that are freaking amazing. It didn't take me long to realize IF is exactly what the woman in her midlife years and beyond needs to melt her midlife middle and live a long, healthy, happy life. Once I began my own Intermittent Fasting journey, I never looked back. In my first year of IF, I released 20 pounds and 20 inches – not only from my midlife middle, but from all over my body. I'm feeling better than I did in my 20's. I am fitting into clothes that are two sizes smaller than when I was at the same weight in my 30's and early 40's. My body has become a fat burning machine, and I have taught women, whose ages range from 42 to 82, to do the same.

I am on a mission to share this information with thousands and thousands of women! I've personally entered a maintenance phase, and I'm finding it effortless because my body has become so efficient. I can't imagine ever going back to the way I used to eat. In truth, my body naturally craved this way of eating, but I resisted because I'd been programmed to believe in the importance of eating three meals a day with snacks in between. I also believed eating was needed for energy before exercising. I should have listened better to my body when I was doing things like forcing myself to drink a morning smoothie because I thought I "should," even though I had no desire or hunger for it whatsoever. My body instinctively KNOWS what is best for me. Why was I resisting? Listening to your body is a BIG part of what I teach when I talk with people about embracing an Intermittent Fasting lifestyle. There are lots of options to adjust Intermittent Fasting to your schedule and personal preferences. Learning what works best for YOU will help you manage your weight easily and achieve long-term success.

This book will walk you through the basic scientific concepts behind Intermittent Fasting, to help you understand WHY all the things you've been doing to lose weight don't work in the short or long term. I'm talking about easy science to explain how fasting helps you become a fat-burning machine like me, so that losing weight and keeping it off becomes effortless. I'll cover why Intermittent Fasting is especially successful for the health and weight management of the midlife woman. We'll explore the ins and outs and how-to's of the 16/8 fasting schedule, including what items are allowed during the fasting parts of the day and what the best food choices are during the eating window. I'll also address using essential oils to boost results. They've been an important part of my own success. I'll review common scenarios you might encounter and their solutions, and will address the concerns and commonly asked questions which I've collected from my clients to help manage the day-to-day Intermittent Fasting lifestyle. In short, I'm going to share EVERYTHING you need to begin your intermittent fasting journey today! Those of you who'd benefit from more interactive, daily support beyond the book to get you started can join my online program called *Melt the Midlife Middle: Eating, Essential Oils & Intermittent Fasting 28 Day Jumpstart Program*. Check out the Resources section for more information.

I don't know about you, but after decades of dealing with the ups and downs of losing and gaining weight, I was tired of it. Tired of thinking about my weight, talking about my weight, and beating myself up about my weight. I never want to weigh or measure another food or count another point again. I just want to live my life, healthy and happy and burden-free from the mental torture my weight has imposed on me all these years. I want the eating freedom to enjoy foods without any guilt or repercussions, and Intermittent Fasting has given me that.

I wrote this book for women everywhere who refuse to let midlife signal the beginning of the end. It is for the women who refuse to resign themselves to the midlife belly and the rocking chair. These are women who feel young and vibrant on the inside, and they want their outside appearance to match. I wrote it for the midlife woman who feels invisible, and wants to not only be noticed again, but to stand out, feel confident, and show the world all the amazing things her life experience has to offer. We have no time to waste! The time is now to regain control of your body, your mind, your health, and to FINALLY lose the stubborn midlife middle once and for all. Here we go!

Chapter 1

Intermittent Fasting At-A-Glance

Who hates the word *diet* as much as I do? Do you know what I see and hear when I look at that word? *DIE-t!* I'd rather do anything than go on another diet. A diet to me is a chore, a forced, unnatural addition outside of your regular daily routine. A diet requires lots of time and effort, both physically and mentally. And when the diet is over, you return to your old ways – thankful that you survived the deprivation. All the work you did just bought you some time until the weight returns, and then you need to start all over again.

Well, that's no longer for me – no way, no how! I got off the diet train years ago by adopting a healthy eating LIFESTYLE. Eighty percent of the time, I ate a clean diet and could indulge the other twenty percent of the time without guilt. I exercised 3 to 5 times a week and was able to maintain a healthy weight for over a decade. But when I entered my mid 40's, that approach to eating stopped working, and the scale kept pointing higher, until I had packed on 20 pounds. . . I got scared. I knew I couldn't do any of the hot, popular diets-of-the-month that are always lurking out there. I knew I couldn't take pills or powders to lose the weight. I really thought I was doomed to carry the extra pounds forever. I needed to find something that would allow me my 80/20 lifestyle AND provide a strategy to release the weight. Intermittent Fasting was what I found – It fit the bill and so much more.

Intermittent Fasting is NOT merely another diet. Intermittent Fasting (IF for short) is a healthy living *lifestyle.* Specifically, Intermittent Fasting is an eating pattern, not based on eating specific foods but instead on WHEN you eat food. You know that saying, "It's either feast or famine?" Well, that's IF in a nutshell.

Now, wait a minute. . . . Don't put the book in the trash because you read the word *famine.* There will be NO deprivation, NO restriction, and NO starvation when you practice IF. There will be periods during the day when you will be eating and periods when you will not. It is as simple, cut and dry as that. You set your own IF schedule and change it up as needed.

A typical day for most Intermittent Fasters ends around 8 PM when they close down the kitchen for the night. They have no after dinner or midnight snacks. Most people are in bed by 10 PM and sleep all night. The majority of the fasting period occurs when they are comfy in their beds sound asleep. IFers wake up in the morning and instead of popping a bagel in the toaster or pouring a big bowl of cereal, which is a habit for most Americans, they stretch the fasting time a few extra hours, enjoying black coffee, unsweetened tea, or inhaling or ingesting essential oils such as lemon or peppermint to help postpone eating a few extra hours. When the clock strikes noon, they open up their eating window for the day without being tied to weighing, measuring, counting, or tracking everything they eat. I teach that you can eat whatever foods you want as long as you are in your eating time window, including sweets and alcohol. You can eat out at restaurants and not be limited to just the salad. You can even have that extra helping!

To be clear, I'm not promoting some free-for-all eating frenzy during a particular time window. It is possible to eat a lot of unhealthy food in eight hours, so there ARE guidelines. I do want you to focus on healthy foods because they are beneficial to you over the long run for your overall health. Eating healthier foods will also make the upcoming fasting period pass much easier. You will feel satisfied longer by eating foods that are higher in fiber and slower to digest. I want you to get results quickly by focusing on eating a balance of foods beginning with healthy fats. Avocados, with 21 grams of healthy fat, are my best friend! Consuming high quality, hormone-free meats and poultry; high fiber (preferably organic) veggies such as broccoli, Brussels sprouts, and carrots; or healthy carbohydrates in moderation such as quinoa can help fill you up and sustain you for many hours.

On the other hand, a cookie or bowl of spaghetti (junk food, unhealthy carbs) is digested quickly, leaving one feeling hungry a mere few hours after eating. When the majority of your meals are comprised of healthy, filling foods, you can work in any treat you want. Are you intrigued by this idea of stretching out the time you don't eat just a little bit so you can really savor, guilt-free, any foods you desire, WHILE losing weight? Are you ready to learn more?

For me, Intermittent Fasting represents eating freedom, it's a way of life, with no endpoint. It's not something that takes over your day, an imposition that overwhelms your thinking and planning. It's not something you "cheat" on. It's not something you are "good" at or "bad" at. It is life! Some days we're on point with eating, and other days we could make better choices. Some days we hit our fasting goals, some days we don't. Sometimes life happens, and we get off course. We don't give up, we just start again the next day. We stick to our fasting schedule and eat well 80% of the time. The other 20% we enjoy, guilt-free, with whatever foods we want, as long as it's in our eating window. It's simple. Simple and freeing.

FASTING IS NOT SOME NEW FAD

Fasting has been used for thousands of years for religious purposes, for spiritual awakening, and for cleansing of the body and mind. There have been periods in history when there wasn't enough food for everyone. People didn't fast by choice but out of necessity. Humans and animals instinctively avoid eating when they don't feel well – a deliberate and unconscious fast. You've seen it, right? Our bodies intuitively know that if we stop eating for a while, our bodies can direct energy toward healing what ails us. We are not meant to be ingesting food all day, every day. Fasting is perfectly natural, and the body not only survives it but can derive some fantastic health benefits from it. Actually, being OVERFED is much more unnatural. Our bodies even have built-in protections specifically for periods of fasting – we store excess fat when we eat, fat that is waiting to be burned to keep us energized and functioning when we need it. This stored fat is our own private energy reserve. A long time ago, men had to hunt for food or they went hungry. Back then, famine was common, and they didn't know when their next meal would come. Their bodies adapted to this lack of food to keep functioning correctly by storing fat to be used later for survival.

We now live in a time when food is literally at our fingertips at any time of day, wherever we are, and we don't need to store fat in fear of the potential famine to come. Unfortunately, our bodies don't know that. We keep eating all day long, and our bodies keep storing what we don't use for energy, and we keep eating, and it keeps storing, and the cycle continues. By never giving our bodies a chance to take a break from eating, we never leave time for the stored fat to be utilized. As stored, unutilized fat fills our cells, we watch our bodies grow larger and larger. Whether we need to lose 50, 75, over a 100 pounds or need to lose those last 5-10 pounds, Intermittent Fasting allows us the time to actually release that stored fat and melt that stubborn midlife middle for good!

We have been socially programmed to eat all day – breakfast, lunch, and dinner with snacks in between. We've heard for years that we need to eat regularly to keep our blood sugar steady, but the result of this way of eating is the fattest, most unhealthy population ever. Incidence of diabetes and obesity is on the rise, even in children. The truth is that eating all day long is doing us no good. Grazing is for cows, NOT for people, and certainly NOT for midlife women!

Chapter 2

The Many Myths Of Weight Loss

I once read a statistic that a woman has tried at least 61 diets by the time she is 45! That is at least two diets per year starting from age 16. That number seemed crazy, and I couldn't find the research to back it, but I'd guess it's probably pretty accurate. Even if you halve that number, it's staggering to remember what we women have been putting ourselves through for most of our lives. And if all the information we have been receiving about how to lose weight was accurate, then why do we need to diet so much? Why can't we lose the weight for good and move on? Well hold on tight, because I am about to throw you off the diet train for good. The information I'm going to share will go against everything you have been told over the years. Be open and receptive to it. Absorb the science supporting your new knowledge. Then experiment for yourself. Nothing beats firsthand results.

MYTH #1

It is inevitable that metabolism slows as you age, making it harder to lose weight.

Metabolism is the process by which your body converts the food you eat (or drink) into energy. Your body needs energy for essential life functions, like breathing, even when you sleep. A *calorie* is a unit of measurement. It is the amount of energy a particular food provides. In other words, it is a way of describing how much energy your body acquires from eating or drinking that food. The number of calories used to keep your body functioning is known as your *basal metabolic rate* (BMR). Think of your BMR as the number of calories (energy) you'd burn lying in bed all day.

Your BMR is determined by your body size and composition (meaning the percentages of fat, bone, water, and muscle), as well as your sex and age. Many people are under another false belief – that as you age, your metabolism slows down. It's an excellent excuse for not losing weight, but it's not exactly true. We will discuss getting older and losing weight in the next chapter, but you should first be aware that it is not necessarily *time* that slows down your BMR. One of the reasons we burn fewer calories as we age is due to the decrease in muscle mass that occurs naturally over time and due to estrogen loss, which consequently slows down the rate at which calories are burned. Many midlife women become more sedentary, decreasing their activity levels as they age, leading to a decline in muscle mass. The more muscle we have, the more efficiently we burn calories. A study called "Regular Exercise and the Age-related Decline in Resting Metabolic Rate in Women" showed that when women regularly do some kind of endurance exercise, such as running or swimming, their metabolism is prevented from slowing down with age. When someone works out consistently, they don't necessarily lose muscle mass. It is totally possible to maintain muscle mass if you're taking care of yourself.

Unfair as it is, men tend to have a faster metabolism than women. That's because men tend to have less body fat and more muscle mass. Men also tend to be taller and bigger overall. If a man has a higher BMR than a woman of the same age, height, and weight, it's because he has more muscle than she does, and thus burns more calories while at rest. Hmm. Could this be a reason that men seem to lose weight easier than women? (Maybe we can forgive them.)

So, how else does our BMR decline? Think about your skinny friend who seems to eat whatever she wants and not gain weight. The false notion is that she has a "high" or "fast" metabolism and easily burns calories. Wrong. In fact, the opposite is true. The more you weigh, the more calories you burn daily. Doesn't your minivan use more gas while idling in the parking lot than your small 2-door car? It's the same concept. Yes, of course there are exceptions to every rule, but just know that the friend you've been cursing for her ability to chow down and never gain weight doesn't possess super metabolism powers. She most likely expends more energy during the day, whether through regular physical activity or the little body movements one doesn't think about such as fidgeting, tapping, and twitching. Or the reason may be plain and simple – your friend restricts their eating or makes healthy choices at other times during the day when you aren't around. I personally get that a lot: People will see me eat 3 of 4 slices of pizza followed by ice cream and ask how I stay so thin. Well, it goes back to my 80/20 rule. They are witnessing only a moment in time. I don't eat like that every day, all day. I strive for balance in my eating choices. My metabolism isn't any faster than anyone else's, and I know this to be accurate because just a year ago I was carrying around 20 extra pounds. Now, in addition to making good choices at least 80% of the time, IF makes it even easier to for me to indulge without significant consequences. I hate to burst your excuse bubble, but your inability to lose weight, especially as you enter midlife, isn't really due to a slow metabolism, even if it's slower than it was 20 years ago.

What is actually happening to your metabolism when you try to lose weight in the traditional model of "Eat Less/ Move More"? I want you to understand that your body is a very smart entity. It works hard to protect itself, maintain proper balance and, like Dr. Jason Fung, author of *The Obesity Code: Unlocking The Secrets Of Weight Loss* and *The Complete Guide To Fasting: Heal Your Body Through Intermittent, Alternate Day and Extended Fasting* writes, "the last thing the body wants to do is die." The results of a 6-year study of *The Biggest Loser* TV show contestants after their season ended suggest reasons why people tend to regain the weight they lose. These TV show contestants used the eat less/move more method, severely restricting their calories while exercising A LOT. They saw their BMR (calories burned at rest) significantly reduced by as much as 800 calories per day – and that BMR didn't recover and reset to where it was, even six years later. This means that after the show ended, they were burning fewer calories during the day. The severe restriction in calories lowered their BMR in what appears to be a lasting change. There has never been a Biggest Loser reunion show, because most contestants stopped the severe food restriction and regained their weight when they went home. This study showed the contestants had lowered their BMR during a prolonged period of food deprivation, and when they started eating more calories, their body only burned the calories to the new, lowered BMR so that the extra calories that were not being burned caused them to regain the weight. My takeaway from this study is the focus for weight loss should not be on restricting calories like most traditional weight loss methods have taught us. I feel the focus should be on helping your body find ways to burn more calories. This can be achieved by eating certain foods, by releasing the stored fat in your cells that's been accumulating in your body over the years, and from exercise. I am describing the Intermittent Fasting lifestyle.

MYTH #2

Breakfast is the most important meal of the day.

I'm all about being an educated consumer, but there are some notions over my lifetime that I bought into without much thought, and one is that breakfast is vital to a healthy diet. Once I understood why that concept was false, and that skipping breakfast would do me no harm, I started to do some research as to where the concept of breakfast's importance originated.

Think for a moment: Who would benefit if breakfast was touted as VITAL to your well-being? Think hard. . . . Perhaps the cereal companies, the dairy industry, and major chicken and pig farmers? Yup. That's right. It was these corporate special interests that spurred the campaign to make "breakfast the most important meal of the day." In fact, they even subsidized "scientific" studies to give their claim credibility. It's no surprise that the studies they funded recommended that every man, woman, and child in the world starts their day with cereal, milk, eggs, and bacon. When I grew up in the seventies, there was a TV commercial that aired during Saturday morning cartoons which recommended a "healthy" breakfast of toast, juice, milk, and a heaping bowl of whatever sugar-laden breakfast cereal they were selling.

Is it any surprise that Americans are fatter than ever? The fact that breakfast is the most important meal of the day simply isn't true. The very term breakfast means to "break a fast," and if you're constantly eating, there's no fast to break. Have you ever heard this adage: "Eat breakfast like a king, lunch like a prince, and dinner like a pauper?" Experts tout the benefits of this morning meal as the revving up your engine needs for the day, a boost to your metabolism. We're taught that eating the morning meal reduces hunger throughout the day. I know I was taught that eating breakfast helps with focus and concentration. In my research to determine whether Intermittent Fasting was good for my body, I discovered breakfast wasn't even considered a particularly meaningful meal until the 19th century. Before then, it was merely a meal like any other. People didn't have specific "breakfast" foods, they would instead eat whatever was lying around or leftovers from dinner the night before, including chicken, steak, or pastries. Our farming ancestors ate a small early meal and a more substantial meal when it was more convenient during the day.

The concept of breakfast as the most important meal of the day was invented in the mid-1800's by Seventh Day Adventists James Caleb Jackson and John Harvey Kellogg to sell their newly invented breakfast cereal. Kellogg was a deeply religious doctor who believed not only that cereal would help improve Americans' health, but also felt that eating red meat created carnal urges, and that cereal would keep people from masturbating and desiring sex. Huh? The Kellogg company, as we know it, was actually created by John's brother Will. Will Kellogg, along with C.W. Post, a former patient whom John Kellogg said stole his recipe, added sugar to John's cereal recipe and took great liberties in their advertising. For example, they claimed it cured malaria and appendicitis and was a good source of Vitamin D. These men were early masters of the art of truth-optional advertising! Cereal became a craze.

This was during the Industrial Revolution, when people were moving to cities where they had less access to kitchens and farms. Cereal was convenient. Soon after, the bacon industry jumped on the bandwagon and convinced people of the importance of eating protein in the morning. Then the dairy guys got in on it. Let's face it – since most people tend to eat the same breakfast most days, manufacturers of breakfast foods have a corner on the market. So in 1944, when the phrase "Breakfast is the most important meal of the day" was coined by the cereal industry, the government-funded nutritionists went along with it by partnering with cereal companies to suggest that everyone eat a "good breakfast of whole-grain cereal and fruit." And there you have it. Government and big business teaming up for mutual benefit. Does that raise any red flags for you??

MYTH #3

One Should Eat Six Small Meals A Day To Lose Weight

How many of us have been told by countless experts and health professionals (including me) that eating three meals and three snacks a day – or six small meals, basically popping food down the hatch every 3 to 4 hours – is necessary if you want to have energy, lose weight, and function properly? That's the mainstream theory. Isn't it interesting to see the rapid increase in obesity over the past 20-30 years? For most of us, it's way too much food. And while it may work for some, Intermittent Fasting science definitely challenges that theory.

Our bodies have two sources for energy: sugar and fat. What is actually going on inside our bodies when we eat? I like to think of the process as a merry-go-round, a carousel. Do you know the Joni Mitchell tune *Carousel*? "And the seasons they go round and round and the painted ponies go up and down, we're captive on a carousel of time. . . ." Well, I made up my own version. Sing it with me: "And the eating cycle goes round and round and our blood sugar goes up and down. We're captives on a carousel of food."

The ride begins when your nose first senses the aroma of food, causing you to salivate. You put the food into your mouth. Yum! A delightful morsel of goodness sends momentary happy signals to the brain. You start to chew, and the carousel begins to move. The digestive process begins as the food carousel moves through the digestive tract where the body efficiently processes, uses, and eliminates what was consumed. You eat again, and the carousel goes round again.

Along the way, your body breaks down everything you eat and absorbs the nutrients. Carbohydrates are broken down by the body and turned into a type of sugar called *glucose,* and our blood sugar level increases. *The painted pony goes up.* Glucose is the primary energy source used by our cells. But here is where the problem starts. Most of us don't stop eating when the body is satisfied. We aren't tuned in to the signals the body is sending. Or maybe we are, and we're just ignoring the messages so we can have that extra piece of birthday cake. The body efficiently uses what energy it can, but if we aren't actively burning off the excess sugar immediately (and after a second piece of cake, I'm betting nothing "active" is happening), the remaining glucose gets converted and stored in the liver temporarily as *glycogen.* At this point, blood sugar levels decrease and then stabilize. *The painted pony comes down, but you don't get off the ride.* Instead, you eat some more and up and down you go again, never giving your body a chance to rest and tap into its stored energy.

MYTH #4

If you want to burn fat, you need to be in ketosis.

A common myth circulating in the media is ketosis is the only way to burn fat. Ketosis occurs when glucose and glycogen stores are depleted and the body turns to fat for energy. Yes, ketosis is one way to put the body into fat burning mode, and it has some great benefits that can be achieved via multiple-day fasting periods or using the Keto diet (a high fat/moderate protein/very low carb diet) but one does NOT need to be in ketosis to burn stored fat.

According to Dr. Eric Berg, DC, advocate for the IF lifestyle and Keto diet, it can take the body 4-6 weeks of fasting or severe carbohydrate restriction for the body to get into a state of full ketosis. Once ketosis is achieved, even one bite of food that contains sugar or starch ends the process and it takes 2-3 days to get back. It is difficult for most people to achieve ketosis regularly unless they are very committed to a highly restrictive diet or willing to do extra-long fasts often. It is a fact that there are many amazing benefits to getting your body into ketosis, but you can still turn your body into a fat burning machine and receive the results you want with shorter fasts, healthy eating and exercise.

I described in Myth #3 how when we are constantly eating, the body is continually processing food, causing blood sugar levels to rise. The high levels of blood sugar signal the release of the fat storing hormone *insulin*, which is essential for stabilizing the blood sugar to return it to a healthy level. It brings blood sugar levels back down by moving glucose out of the bloodstream and into storage as fat. On the other hand, when blood sugar levels are low, *glucagon* (not to be confused with glycogen or glucose) is released. Glucagon signals the release of stored fat back into the bloodstream so that it can be used for fuel. When glucagon is released, the body taps into the stored fat and burns it for energy, without being in full ketosis.

Intermittent Fasting is one way to trigger glucagon. The body quickly adapts to burning stored fat when consistently living an IF lifestyle. Before the body becomes a proficient fat burner, most people start to feel hungry and depleted when their blood sugar and insulin levels get low (usually 10-12 hours into a fast). This is usually when they pop something into their mouth to curb the cravings. When the body becomes proficient at fat burning, hunger will still be felt, but you won't feel "hangry" (irritability coming from perceived hunger – anger + hungry = hangry), and you'll be able to easily extend the fasting time. The glucagon kicks in, and now there is plenty of energy for the body. This glucagon release is the "money shot." It's pure fat burning gold!

Three ways to trigger glucagon release are Intermittent Fasting (allowing your body the time to let insulin levels get low), Keto Diet (a diet high in healthy fats and low in processed carbs), and exercise. I do not personally choose to participate in a Keto diet. It is too restrictive for me. I'd rather eat less often, but eat the foods I enjoy when I do eat – which IF allows – rather than deprive myself of my favorite foods. When exercising, the body releases endorphins, which in turn cause a release of glucagon, making exercise one of the easiest, most effective ways to increase the body's ability to burn stored fat. Exercise also builds up muscle mass and increases the number of calories burned at rest. Now that's a great reason to hit the gym!

Fasting long enough to get into and stay in true ketosis may not be realistic for everyone, but exercising and limiting the number of times a day the body spikes insulin is entirely doable, and yet another reason why the Intermittent Fasting lifestyle just makes sense.

If you just take one thing away from all this science, make it this: The body CANNOT store and release fat at the same time. Eating causes the release of insulin, which is a FAT STORING hormone. Periods of fasting trigger the release of glucagon, which is a STORED FAT RELEASING hormone. Again: *It is IMPOSSIBLE for the body to store and release fat at the same time.* Eating every 3 to 4 hours prevents fat release and promotes fat storage. MIC DROP MOMENT! It's suddenly clear why eating throughout the day is counterproductive to losing that stubborn belly fat and why my middle-aged clients had difficulty losing weight despite their best efforts. It's not because the fat is stubborn, it's us! When you're constantly eating throughout the day, you're on the carousel ride from hell – not only can you never get off, but your jeans keep getting tighter and tighter. Isn't it time to get off the eating carousel and try something new?

MYTH #5

You shouldn't work out on an empty stomach.

Since most people doing IF are skipping breakfast, one of the first concerns people raise is whether they can safely and effectively work out during the fasting state. The answer is a resounding YES! This was originally my top concern, since I run and do weight training and prefer to work out in the morning. I have found that since I've been doing IF, I have tons of energy during my workouts with no dizziness or other issues. Unless you find yourself getting lightheaded during a fast, feel free to exercise to your heart's content – cardio, weightlifting, the works. "Several elite-level strength athletes have told me that their strength peaks after a 16- or 20-hour fast," writes Dr. Dominic D'Agostino, Ph.D., at the University of South Florida Health. "Cognitively, people tend to feel more lucid and focused. The more frequently you fast the easier it gets and the more benefits you'll derive from it." He continues, "The most important thing to consider for people who do intermittent fasting, whether it is 14 hours or 16 hours from dinner until the first meal the next day, is what the first meal of the day is and how that fits into your exercise schedule." He adds that "it is important to eat protein, complex carbs, healthy fats, and plant-rich fibers during the eating window to maintain a healthy fast. More complex carbs are needed for workout days. More protein, plant fibers, and fats are needed on rest days." Many clients of mine, including marathon runners, cyclists, and morning exercisers, were worried at first about how their performance would be affected by Intermittent Fasting. Shortly after committing to IF, they discovered that not only could they easily perform their workout on an empty stomach, but that they also felt more energized, had increased endurance, and didn't feel the need to eat right after finishing.

There are enormous benefits to exercising while in a fasted state, especially for the middle-aged woman. They include:

1. **Exercising in a fasted state burns more stored fat.** Research shows that if you work out before, rather than after eating breakfast in the morning, you can burn nearly 20% more fat. Once we eat, insulin increases in the body. According to some research, higher insulin levels have been shown to suppress fat burning by up to 22 percent. You'd need to do a whole lot of exercise to overcome that!

2. **Fasted exercise can also help those extra pounds from coming on when you overindulge.** In one 6-week study, researchers asked volunteers to pig out on junk food every day. Some volunteers didn't exercise at all, others fasted before working out in the morning, and others ate a big breakfast before working out. Results showed that those in the first group who overate and didn't exercise gained the most weight. Makes sense. Those who ate breakfast before a workout also gained weight, about half as much as the first group. Hmmm. The subjects who exercised during their fast gained virtually no weight, even though they ate just as poorly. I am definitely not promoting gorging on junk food, but I do appreciate the fact that the participants who fasted before breakfast gained no weight.

3. **Exercise increases insulin sensitivity.** A resistance to insulin (low insulin sensitivity) is what causes metabolic syndrome (aka pre-diabetes), which many midlife women experience. In the study described above, after piling on the junk food, both the non-exercisers and the non-fasting exercisers exhibited increased resistance to insulin, while the fasted exercisers showed no signs of insulin resistance despite their poor eating. In another study, participants exercised in a fasted state at least 3 times a week. At the end of 12 weeks, they lost an average of ¼ of their baseline fat mass, and their fasting insulin levels fell by 25%!

4. **Athletic performance increases when you exercise while fasting.** Up until now, your body has been trained to treat sugar, not fat, as its primary energy source. You are carrying around all this stored fat that's ready to serve its purpose of providing you with energy, yet you have no way of tapping into it. Often, during a hard workout, you may feel that your body can't do any more and that you're "hitting the wall." This occurs because you've burned through all the sugar, but your body's not efficient at accessing the stored fat. Fasting can help you access the stored fat and become a fat burning machine – combine fasting with exercise and watch your endurance and results soar.

5. **Exercise increases the production of Human Growth Hormone (HGH)**, AKA the "fountain of youth," which unfortunately diminishes with age. HGH helps the body build new muscle tissue, burn fat, improve bone quality (an issue for aging women), and increase longevity. Along with regular strength training and proper sleep, fasting is one of the best ways to increase the body's amount of HGH. Stay

tuned for more on this crucial hormone for the midlife woman in the next chapter.

I hope you are starting to realize that there is hope for losing the midlife middle for good, and that Intermittent Fasting might just be the thing you have been searching for all this time.

Chapter 3

Why Is It So Hard For Women To Lose The Midlife Middle?

Now that you understand the basic physiology behind IF, let's look at how it has impacted the lives of some real women.

Joy, 48, played tennis, did yoga a few times a week, and tried to eat healthfully. In spite of her best efforts, her waistline kept expanding. Although she was unhappy with her appearance, she wasn't willing to give up the foods she loved and a lifestyle that including eating out and occasionally indulging with some wine and dessert. "I am self-employed and always super busy. In the past, I would grab whatever was close by when I had a chance. Since starting IF 5 months ago, my whole palette has changed. Not only am I easily able to fast 16-18 hours a day, but I no longer crave a lot of the junk food I had been eating. Because I only have a set time of eating, I make sure I only eat foods I love. No more cheap burgers for me – give me the filet mignon!"

Maya, 51, was completely beside herself. Once a size 4, she was having trouble fitting into size 12, and it was seriously hurting her self-esteem. Despite a healthy, plant-based diet and regular exercise, she couldn't control her weight.

"Intermittent Fasting made a world of sense to me from the start. I researched and watched a ton of videos and then connected with Jill and her *Melt the Midlife Middle* program. I realized that as important as the fasting is, it is equally important that when you do eat, you eat well – healthy, satisfying, nutrient-rich meals and without deprivation. The weight is starting to come off, and my pants are getting looser. IF has helped me start feeling good about myself again."

At this point, I hope you understand why I am so excited about IF and the possibilities it holds for so many women who want to melt the midlife middle. But let's jump into why IF works so well for losing belly fat and increasing vitality and longevity, specifically for a woman in her midlife years and beyond.

As you've entered the midlife years, have you found your waistline expanding? Have you wondered why it is so hard to lose weight since you hit your mid 40's? It's because what the body needs at 20 and 30 is different than what it needs at 50 and 60 years old. Dr. Stephanie S. Faubion, Mayo Clinic physician and author of the book "*The Menopause Solution*", teaches that weight gain during midlife is common, and that about two-thirds of women ages 40 to 59 are overweight. She says that "on average, midlife women gain 1.5 pounds per year." Dr. Faubion writes, "Obesity, and specifically abdominal obesity, increases the risk of chronic medical conditions in post-menopausal women, including diabetes, hypertension, hyperlipidemia, certain cancers (including breast and uterine cancers), and heart disease, the number-one killer of women." Dr. Faubion continues, "Women who are obese may also experience more severe hot flashes. In addition, there is an emotional burden related to weight gain in midlife that can affect a woman's self-image, relationship with her partner, and even her sexual function."

Dr. Faubion gives excellent reasons to once and for all get to a healthy and fit version of yourself. My book, "*No Sweat! It's Just Menopause: Eating Exercise & Essential Oils For A Healthy Change*" goes into detail about much of the science behind menopause in an easy and digestible way. I recommend reading it or getting educated on menopause from a different reliable source. Knowledge is power, and it will help you to take control of your well-being and ease yourself through this stage of life.

There are different reasons the midlife woman gains weight, especially in the midsection, and why she has such a hard time losing it. A decline in estrogen production is at the top of the list.

ESTROGEN DECLINE

Estrogen has over 400 functions. Do you think that if something was messing with our estrogen levels, we might feel some fallout? Definitely!

According to an article from the Endocrine Society's Hormone Health Network your body makes three main types of estrogen:

Estradiol (E2): the most common type in women of childbearing age

Estriol (E3): the main estrogen during pregnancy

Estrone (E1): the only estrogen your body makes after menopause (once menstrual periods stop)

Estradiol production specifically decreases at menopause. This is an important hormone for managing a woman's weight and metabolism. Some experts feel that lower levels of estradiol may lead to weight gain. During her teen years and throughout her 20's and 30's, a woman tends to gain weight around her hips and thighs. After menopause, that distribution changes. The weight gain shifts to her entire midsection. This type of fat is different than the love handles we can see and touch. This kind of fat hits the belly and the surrounding organs and is known as *visceral* fat. You want to avoid this kind of fat, because visceral fat can be very damaging. It has been linked to heart disease, stroke, diabetes, and some cancers. A lack of estrogen may also cause the body to be less efficient in converting blood sugars into energy. This leads to more fat being stored and makes it harder to lose weight.

WE MOVE LESS AS WE AGE

Although some researchers have concluded that there is a connection between decreased estrogen production and weight gain, others have found that weight gain does not appear to be affected by hormonal changes related to menopause. A review of studies from 2012, titled "Understanding Weight Gain at Menopause," concluded that menopause may not be the worst weight gain culprit, and that gaining weight in the midlife years can instead be attributed to a decline in lean muscle mass and a decrease in activity level.

Well, I certainly understand the decline in activity level. Women in their midlife years, particularly those going through menopause, have a whole bunch of annoyances including night sweats, sleep disturbance, and mood issues. Who the heck feels like going to the gym when you already look and feel like a hot mess?! Also, many midlife women are part of the "sandwich" generation. They are sandwiched between taking care of their kids and their own aging parents, not to mention their husbands, their bosses, and all the other obligations they take on, all of which lead to extra stress. Combine that with hormonal changes, and of course all you want to do is lie on the couch, eat your favorite Ben & Jerry's ice cream, and veg out in front of the TV. If you aren't sleeping well, you might turn to quick sugar boosts for your energy, like candy bars or other unhealthy snacks that also add weight to your midsection. You may be dealing with physical limitations – such as knee pain or back issues – and can't do traditional exercise. Certain medications (including antidepressants, which are commonly prescribed to midlife women) can also promote weight gain. In *"No Sweat! It's Just Menopause"*, I list some natural alternatives to help you get a good night's sleep, manage muscle and joint discomfort, and improve your emotional well-being.

LEAN MUSCLE MASS

In Chapter 2, I said most women begin to lose lean body mass as a result of the normal aging process and a decrease in estrogen production that occurs during midlife. If you recall, a reduction in lean muscle mass ends up slowing down the rate at which you burn calories. The more muscle we have, the more efficiently we burn calories. Lean muscle mass helps us to burn calories, so when it decreases – either because we're slowing down and are not as active or due to decreased estrogen levels as we enter perimenopause and full menopause – we burn fewer calories both at rest and when we exercise. The midlife woman should find a nice balance between exercises that increase heart rate and those that are muscle building, as well as exercises for flexibility, balance, and mental relaxation. Chapter 7 gives you details about the best exercises for the midlife woman.

HUMAN GROWTH HORMONE

We've also touched upon the Human Growth Hormone (HGH), and I promised to tell you more about this fantastic hormone that can help you to look and feel younger. HGH levels affect our lean muscle mass, much as estrogen does. HGH is a naturally occurring hormone produced by the pituitary gland. It plays a vital role in human growth and the regeneration and reproduction of cells in the body. HGH helps to maintain, build, and repair healthy tissue in the brain and other organs. This hormone can help speed up the healing process after an injury, and can repair muscle tissue after exercise. For our weight loss needs, HGH helps to build muscle mass, boost metabolism, and burn fat. HGH is also just what aging skin needs. It helps us keep up a youthful appearance. It plays a role in helping the midlife woman continue to look and feel young on the outside and inside, as well as combat illnesses that commonly occur as one ages. You get serious bang for your buck with this hormone!

Let's look at HGH in terms of eating and fasting. When you eat, the release of the human growth hormone is restricted by the rise of insulin in your system. Research cardiologists at the Intermountain Medical Center Heart Institute have found that routine periodic fasting is good for your health and your heart. They discovered that after a 24-hour fast, HGH production in females increased by 1,300%. This is thought to occur due to the body's effort to protect its lean muscle mass and other metabolic functions. Some of my IF clients are noticing an interesting side effect of fasting 16 hours daily. They're starting to look YOUNGER! Sure, weight loss can make us look more youthful, but it's more than that. The changes in their hair, skin and nails make sense because of the enormous increase in HGH they're experiencing. Who'd ever think that fasting could be the difference between called "Ma'am" and "Miss" in the grocery store? One client told me that after several months of IF, she is once again "Miss" one hundred percent of the time!

The more estrogen we women have circulating, the more human growth hormone we produce. As we age and enter menopause, our estrogen supply dramatically decreases, and therefore so does our production of HGH. HGH is also thought to raise *testosterone* levels, which also deplete with age. Testosterone isn't just a male hormone – it plays a crucial role in the development and maintenance of muscle mass, strength, energy levels, and bone density for both sexes. For women in particular, the maintenance of bone density and muscle mass is essential, as both of these tend to deteriorate with age. Testosterone can also boost libido.

Between the estrogen drop, testosterone drop, and the drop in HGH production, you can see why the midlife woman needs to do what she can to raise her HGH levels. And fasting and exercise both help to do just that. It makes sense to conclude that a combination of working out regularly and adopting an Intermittent Fasting lifestyle could accelerate results.

Some other potential benefits of adequate HGH for women are:

- Relieves chronic anxiety
- Allows the body to function optimally even with less sleep
- Helps to reduce the buildup of fat in the abdominal area, the knees, and in the hips
- Helps to strengthen the body
- Helps a woman to keep her natural shape

STRESS

Another factor against us in our fight to release fat is *stress.* Due to the many obligations the midlife woman has mentioned above, stress becomes a significant factor in the midlife woman's ability to lose that stubborn fat.

In addition to converting the carbohydrates we ingest to sugars (glucose), when the body is under stress, it releases the hormone *cortisol*. Cortisol produces sugar made from proteins in the liver. It increases the amount of glucose the body can store so that it can rapidly increase its energy in times of stress, which is vital for those truly threatening "fight or flight" moments when the body needs the extra boost. Living in a constant state of stress makes the body produce more sugars. In a study led by Dr. Sarah Jackson and published in the journal "Obesity," she determined that high levels of cortisol due to chronic stress increases the risk of obesity, particularly in the midsection. The stored fat from excess cortisol is the visceral fat I mentioned above. It is hard to get rid of. Abdominal fat cells are very sensitive to high insulin levels, and they are excellent at storing fat because they're so close to your digestive organs. This is another reason why women develop that midlife middle that just won't budge.

In addition to cortisol's release as a response to outside stressors, another factor that can cause overproduction and imbalance in cortisol levels is the overconsumption of simple carbs, like those found in candy bars or soda. I've already explained how insulin is released to lower the blood sugar spikes we experience when we eat these foods. This same up-and-down pattern of insulin, glucose, and cortisol levels either doesn't occur or is significantly less dramatic when one eats a balanced diet of fats, proteins, fiber, and complex carbohydrates (such as quinoa), because the processes of digestion and absorption are slowed down. In Chapter 5, I will cover ways to eat healthy for optimal body functioning.

TOXIC OVERLOAD

There's one other major factor that may contribute to midlife women's hormonal imbalance and her stubborn midsection that's so difficult to lose. It's the exposure to toxic chemicals we encounter daily – and sometimes unknowingly – all day long, in small doses from the environment, from the dry cleaners, from the personal care products we use daily. Toxins such as parabens and phthalates are commonly found in our cosmetics and cleaning products that are fragranced. Toxic exposure from these products accumulates over time, causing serious issues that impact the body's functioning. Our cells get all gunked up with these man-made chemicals. Miscommunication happens at the cellular level in the body, and problems develop, including obesity, cancers, and Alzheimer's Disease. Then there are secondary issues – not quite as dramatic, but still annoying and which affect your life – like poor sleeping, decreased energy, no sex drive, wrinkles, hair loss, and hot flashes.

This toxic exposure really speeds up the aging process. The body has no need for this cellular junk, so it just sits in our cells wreaking havoc until it's expelled through some method of detoxification. Natural ways to purge these toxins include Intermittent Fasting and essential oils. In Chapter 4, we will talk about essential oils and how they can help.

AUTOPHAGY

What if I told you that in addition to burning fat and increasing HGH, Intermittent Fasting also helps you get rid of the toxic gunk stored in your cells? Did your ears perk up? If not, they should because you will want to understand this next impressive benefit of IF called *autophagy* (pronounced "o-TAWF-uh-gee"). The 2016 Nobel Prize in Physiology or Medicine was awarded to Yoshinori Ohsumi for his research on autophagy. It refers to the way the cells clean themselves by removing toxins and other waste. If we never allow our body to reach autophagy, the cellular buildup of toxins continues. Naomi Whittel, *author of Glow15: A Science Based Plan to Lose Weight, Revitalize Your Skin and Invigorate Your Life, wrote:* "when autophagy is in play, your cells eat away at the junk, removing and recycling the waste that leads to the visible signs of aging." "Think of it as our body's innate recycling program," says Colin Champ, M.D., a board-certified radiation oncologist, assistant professor at the University of Pittsburgh Medical Center, and author of *Misguided Medicine.* He writes, "Autophagy makes us more efficient machines to get rid of faulty parts, stop cancerous growths, and stop metabolic dysfunction like obesity and diabetes."

As we get older, like so many other things, the autophagy process becomes less efficient. It requires a little boost for optimal functioning. An easy way to make this happen is to take a 12+ hour timeout from food consumption. Give your body's cells and tissues the time they need to clean themselves, and you should see and feel the positive changes. When we eat or drink, the hormone insulin, as we have learned, is automatically released to balance blood sugar levels. As we covered in the previous chapter, the opposite process occurs when in a fasting state: The cells have a break from processing foods, insulin levels decrease, and when insulin levels fall too low, glucagon is released. When we fast for more than 12 hours, this glucagon increase not only triggers fat burning but also triggers autophagy. Fasting for more than 12 hours at a time is one of the best ways to rejuvenate our cells by cleaning them of the toxic goop, which slows (and possibly reverses) the aging process. I don't know about you, but I am more than willing to give up food for a few extra hours to turn back the hands of time.

NON-WEIGHT RELATED BENEFITS OF FASTING

A study came out in April 2016 in the *Journal of Mid-Life Health,* titled "The Role of Therapeutic Fasting in Women: An Overview." It revealed many exciting things about the positive impact fasting can have on women's wellness. One, it concluded that fasting was successful for reducing belly fat in older women. It also revealed that fasting had many non-weight benefits, including improved reproductive and mental health. It also prevents cancers and improves musculoskeletal disorders, which are common in middle-aged and elderly women. Fasting improved women's muscle and joint pain. Also, low back pain and arthritis was less noticeable.

The study revealed that there was even some possible link to periods of fasting and improved bone health. For many women, osteoporosis becomes an issue as we age, so anything we can do to strengthen our bones is good. The study also showed that "fasting led to the slowing down of cancer growth and even blocked pathways to develop cancers." And in terms of mental health, anxiety and depression seemed to lessen, whereas mood and confidence improved. That's a serious plug for Intermittent Fasting! The study reported no adverse side effects of fasting, only that more testing is needed to learn more about beneficial effects.

SELF-PERCEPTION

Mirror mirror on the wall, who's the fattest of them all? For so many women body image is linked to self-worth and self-confidence. When some women look in the mirror, negative feelings arise that have often existed since childhood. For some, these feelings about their body may date back to watching and listening to their mothers and grandmothers, seeing and hearing how they viewed their bodies. Growing up, they witnessed these women they loved calling themselves an "elephant," refusing to wear a bathing suit, not allowing people to take their photo, ridiculing others for being overweight. These early observations no doubt stuck in their mind.

Although unintentional, our early role models created within us a subconscious connection between outward appearance and intrinsic worth. Our moms aren't the only ones to blame about how we view ourselves. Some women have experienced bullying in school due to their weight, or perhaps a well-intentioned loved one made a remark about their appearance that was hurtful. Society piggybacks on these feelings of insecurity with its love affair with anything young, beautiful, and thin. Beauty and cosmetic sales are soaring these days with no end in sight. *Forbes* magazine reports the beauty industry is a $445 billion dollar market! Women compare themselves to an impossible standard (truly impossible: the photos in today's magazines are nearly all Photoshopped) and feel they come up short.

When we think negatively about what we see in the mirror, we begin to live behind the scenes in the movie of our lives. How we feel about our body holds us back from pursuing our dream job, becoming sex goddesses in the bedroom, or standing up and speaking our mind – to those who treat us poorly, or to those who may need our wisdom. We hold back the unique gifts we were put on this earth to share with others, and all because of some excess flesh hanging over our jeans. It seems crazy, but it's true.

For me, Intermittent Fasting changed so much more than the shape of my body – it transformed me on the inside. Being in control of my eating has helped me feel in control of my life again. For some time, I was letting life happen TO me, feeling like a loser, annoyed by my own negative thoughts. As the pounds I had accumulated melted away, I found myself releasing the heavy energy that burdened me.

SEX & INTIMACY

For many women, success with IF brings out their inner lioness between the sheets. Many midlife women tell me their libidos are shot, sex is uncomfortable, and they are embarrassed to be seen naked. Many midlife women tell me they haven't had sex with their partner in months, even years. I asked a question on my Facebook page, "What is more important to you: having great sex or losing weight?" Overwhelmingly, the responses were, "If I lost the weight, the sex would get better, and I would want it more." And believe me, it is true! When you feel good about yourself, that shows up in all areas of your life, and a hot sex life is what I call a non-scale victory. Yay for Intermittent Fasting!

The midlife woman faces declining estrogen, a decrease in lean muscles mass, and less production of HGH as she ages, all of which contribute to stubborn belly fat that seems impossible to lose. Many women give up trying to lose weight because it feels like such an uphill battle. IF can be the long-awaited solution. Intermittent Fasting is an excellent way of eating that holds specific benefits for the midlife woman. Intermittent Fasting not only helps us lose the belly fat, it also slows down the aging process through the increased production of HGH and the process of autophagy. IF improves energy levels, bone health, mental clarity, and emotional distress.

Did you ever think that not eating could have so many positive side effects? What are your feelings about skipping breakfast at this point now that you have learned about all the incredible benefits you will reap just for saying "not now, later" to your eggs and bacon? Are you ready to jump on my IF bandwagon? I hope it is a resounding YES! YES! YES!

Chapter 4

Essential Oils & Intermittent Fasting- A Recipe For Success

There are six common essential oils I use to help me with Intermittent Fasting, and you'll want to be sure to have all of them in your cupboard. To make this IF recipe for success, you'll need the following essential oils: Grapefruit, Lemon, Peppermint, Bergamot, Cinnamon, and Ginger. I personally use Young Living essential oils (see *Resources*), including oils from their Vitality line which are labeled safe for ingestion. If you use other essential oils that are not created by Young Living, please do your due diligence and check to make sure they are high quality oils that won't harm you when used internally.

When people think of essential oils, they often think of how pretty the oil smells. But quality essential oils go far beyond just pleasing your sense of smell. Essential oils can support your physical, emotional, hormonal, and sexual well-being, areas needing an extra boost in the life of the midlife woman. When I embarked upon my own IF journey, I had already been using essential oils in all those areas, as well as for years to cook with, put in my smoothies, and flavor my water. I knew that many oils supported healthy weight and metabolism and helped to curb food cravings. I also knew that some oils could be cleansing for the body. Combining IF and essential oils for me was a no brainer. I knew they would be powerful together, and I was right. Essential oils can support you during the times you are eating, as well as the times you are not eating when doing IF.

MIDLIFE WOMEN & TOXIC OVERLOAD

Essential oils have been around since biblical times but recently have had a resurgence in popularity due to people being sick of feeling ill and tired all the time. Women are realizing that all the toxins and chemicals they knowingly (and unknowingly) expose themselves to on a daily basis, in culprits such as detergents, cleaners, makeup, sprayed pesticides, processed foods, medicines, and air pollution are a contributing factor to many of the physical and emotional issues they are having, and they want a natural alternative. Many of these issues disrupt their daily lives. Poor digestion, trouble falling or staying asleep, and skin breakouts are a few minor but annoying problems. There are much bigger problems that occur with overexposure to chemicals, such as a higher likelihood of a breast cancer diagnosis. According to a review by the SEER program, which provides cancer statistics for the National Institute for Health's National Cancer Institute, "Rates for new female breast cancer cases have been rising on average .3% each year over the last 10 years." The statistics collected show that more than half of women diagnosed in the US have no known risk factors. Only 10% of the women diagnosed with breast cancer have a family history with the disease.

In the past year, three of my friends, all in their 40's, have been diagnosed with breast cancer. None of them had a family history, and they all lived a healthy lifestyle the best they could. I'm sure almost everyone reading this book knows someone who has fought breast cancer. If there is no family history or risk factors, then why are so many women stricken with this disease? Many of the toxins we're exposed to daily have been linked to women's cancers, especially those we're exposed to before entering full menopause. Toxins also increase a woman's risk of heart disease, as stated earlier, the #1 killer of women over 50. This toxic overload from the foods we eat, the products we use, and the air we breathe may result in midlife women gaining weight that is difficult to release, having low energy, crazy moods, and reduced sex drive. Many midlife women already feel like hot messes due to changing hormones, and now we have to worry about chemicals in our makeup and pesticides on our salads? Enough!

ALL OILS ARE NOT CREATED EQUALLY

Essential oils are Mother Nature's little drops of goodness. They are extracted from all parts of plants, trees, flowers, seeds, and citrus rind, and they are either steam distilled or cold pressed. It is important to note that not all oils are created equal. This is especially important if you choose to ingest oils. READ YOUR OIL LABELS!! Most oils on the market have been adulterated in some way to cut corners, save money, and yield more oil faster. These oils have had alcohol or solvents mixed with them, or have been distilled (the action of purifying a liquid by a process of heating and cooling) at high temperatures to move the product to the shelves quicker, sacrificing the natural benefits of that oil. Oils distilled at low temperatures maintain the integrity of the oil. Most oils on the market come from genetically modified seeds, or are grown in "dirty" soil with the help of harmful fertilizers or sprayed pesticides. Why in the world, if you're trying to lessen your toxic exposure, would you want to use oils that were compromised? It completely defeats the purpose. Knowing the source of your essential oils is the

41

key to knowing whether it is pure, chemical-free, and made by a company that adheres to strict growing and reaping standards. Be an educated consumer when using essential oils, especially when using them for a purpose, as with Intermittent Fasting. Don't just throw one in your cart when out shopping at the drug store because you like the price tag – the true cost of using a cheap oil may be paid by your body.

WHY ESSENTIAL OILS ARE EFFECTIVE

Let's talk a little oily science for a moment. Essential oils are made up of thousands of chemical compounds. The most important ones are *phenols, monoterpenes,* and *sesquiterpenes*.

Phenols have antioxidant properties, and they clean receptor sites of cells so that sesquiterpenes can delete misinformation written on the DNA of the cell. This misinformation that shows up as physical problems or disease is a result of our cells being clogged up with toxic gunk. These toxins, when absorbed through our skin, breathed, or ingested, take up residence in our cells and fester there unless we intentionally do something – like detoxification – to remove them from our body. If the toxins just sit there, they cause problems and miscommunication between the cells so that the body doesn't function properly. Some of these toxins have an estrogen-like quality that interacts with our body, putting us in a state of hormonal flux. After the phenols and sesquiterpenes have done their job, the monoterpenes then correct and rewrite the information in the DNA of the cell. Monoterpenes and sesquiterpenes are present in nearly all essential oils.

In the previous chapter, we discussed the process of autophagy, the cleansing of the cells, that's typically induced after 12 hours of fasting. Do you see how combining Intermittent Fasting and reaching autophagy, combined with using essential oils to attack toxins, can be like hitting the cell cleaning jackpot?! And when our cells are clean, healthy, and working as they should, our success with IF can soar.

HOW TO USE ESSENTIAL OILS

There are three ways to use essential oils to make Intermittent Fasting easier and support a healthy lifestyle. You feel their effects physically within minutes of use.

Inhalation: Inhale the scent right from the bottle, or put a few drops in a cold air diffuser and let the aroma fill the room to uplift mood. Breathing in the scent can keep your focus on making good, healthy food choices or holding out a little longer before breaking the fast with food.

Topical: Essential oils can be used on the skin. It is best to combine 1-2 drops with a couple of teaspoons of carrier oil, either in a small bowl or in a glass roll-on with a stainless steel top. Carrier oils are fat-based oils such as coconut oil, grapeseed oil, and jojoba oil that slow the absorption of the essential oil into the skin so it can be spread on the skin more easily. The carrier oils also dilute the essential oil to prevent any skin reaction. Should a reaction occur, add more carrier oil by itself directly to the skin. Essential oils used topically can provide digestive support as new foods are added to the diet, as well as promote smooth, youthful skin.

Ingestion: Essential oils labeled safe for ingestion can be consumed internally to add flavor, act as a daily cleanse, energize, or relax the body and mind and support the immune system. Essential oils are simple to use and cost effective, especially for cooking. You know how a recipe will call for just a tablespoon of fresh rosemary, but you have to buy the whole bunch and the rest gets thrown out, wasting food and money? When you substitute essential oils for fresh herbs and spices, you will only need 1-2 drops or even less. When adding strong oils like oregano, you will need to dip a toothpick in the oil and swirl it into whatever you are cooking. The end of this chapter provides rules for cooking with essential oils and suggestions to incorporate them into your kitchen.

MY TOP SIX ESSENTIAL OIL PICKS FOR INTERMITTENT FASTING SUCCESS

The first group of oils is from the citrus family. Citrus oils contain high amounts of *limonene,* which is both an antioxidant and a monoterpene. It is found in the rinds of citrus fruits. Registered dietician, Staci Shacter, MS, RD, LDN, says that compounds like d-limonene help to "support your metabolism and cleanse your lymphatic glands so they can carry nutrients between the tissues and the bloodstream." An article coming out of the University of Bristol noted that "limonene constitutes 98% (by weight) of the essential oil obtained from the orange peel." Limonene is helpful for the Intermittent Faster.

Grapefruit Oil

Close your eyes and pretend you've just cut open a fresh grapefruit off the tree. You can almost taste the tangy, bitter, yet refreshing flavor. You get the same sensation when you take a whiff of 100% pure Grapefruit oil. Grapefruit essential oil contains 86-92% d-limonene and is highly concentrated when distilled from the grapefruit. The properties of grapefruit have been significantly researched. Who has tried the Grapefruit Diet? It has been around for years, and it turns out it's not a myth. The research by the Nutrition and

Metabolic Research Center at Scripps Clinic pointed toward a physiological link between grapefruit and insulin related to weight management. The results of the study indicated that the "chemical properties of grapefruit reduce insulin levels and encourage weight loss." And as we have already seen, the fewer insulin spikes we have, the more efficiently our bodies utilize energy from foods and the less fat that needs to be stored.

Shacter also says, "There is a ton of research showing how eating grapefruit helps promote weight loss by helping with blood sugar, appetite, and the breakdown of fat. . . . Grapefruit essential oil has been shown to impact the same mechanisms for weight loss as eating grapefruit." Grapefruit essential oil helps to activate enzymes in the body that work to break down body fat. Studies also show that using grapefruit oil "affects autonomic nerves, which regulate important body functions like heart rate and digestion, and reduce appetite and body weight."

Grapefruit can also be a cosmetic boost during weight loss efforts. Think smooth, non-dimply skin. *According to the International Journal of Cosmetic Science,* "the primary way grapefruit can be used to reduce cellulite is through inhaling the vapor of the extract because it stimulates the nervous system 250%." That sounds like aromatherapy to me. Grapefruit also contains skin cleansing properties including an enzyme, bromelain, that's known to help break down cellulite.

There are three ways – inhaling, topical application, and ingestion – that the grapefruit oil can be used to support a healthy weight. Adding grapefruit oil to a vegetable capsule or in your water, or combining it with some coconut oil and rubbing it on your skin, or taking a few big inhales may support the body in similar ways to the eating the actual fruit. **Grapefruit has been known to interact with some**

medications, especially blood pressure medication, so check with your doctor before using if this applies to you.

Lemon Oil

If you've been on the diet train for a long time, then you've probably heard of using lemon water to lose weight and detoxify your body. You may have tried it and had success, but it isn't always convenient because we don't usually carry lemons on us. Lemon essential oil is easy to transport, 1-3 drops is all you need, so you can drink lemon water no matter where you are. Lemon essential oil as compared to lemon juice is not acidic. Meaning that unlike lemon juice, the oil doesn't damage teeth enamel. Lemon, another citrus oil, is also high in d-limonene, Vitamin C, and other minerals which can help support digestion, detoxification of the fat cells, and a healthy metabolism. In a study in the *Journal of Clinical Biochemistry and Nutrition,* mice were put on a fattening diet and given "lemon polyphenols extracted from the peel." They gained less weight and body fat than other mice. This study hasn't been performed on humans yet, but it sounds promising! I've had many clients break through their weight loss plateaus, doing nothing different other than adding a few drops of lemon oil to their water. Their results made me a believer!

Plus, staying hydrated is an integral part of a healthy diet. Drinking lots of water helps you feel full during the fasting stage of your day. Flavoring your water with lemon oil may help you to drink more, especially if you struggle drinking plain water.

I also love adding lemon essential oil to my diffuser to increase my energy and improve my mood. I was excited to learn from the research that breathing in the scent of lemon essential oil improves the neurological activity that promotes the breakdown of body fat. BONUS!

Peppermint

There is something about the taste of peppermint that is cool, clean, and refreshing. It brings up fond memories for me of eating candy canes, peppermint patties, and peppermint stick ice cream. Peppermint is my favorite essential oil because of its versatility. I use it in numerous ways daily, from putting it in a spray bottle with water as a cooling spray when exercising or having a hot flash, using it as a breath freshener, and for keeping me awake and alert when driving.

Peppermint has the tested scientific research to back it up. Based on their own research, the agency Organic Facts concluded that peppermint oil is packed with minerals and nutrients such as "manganese, iron, magnesium, calcium, folate, potassium, and copper. It also contains Omega 3 fatty acids, Vitamin A and Vitamin C, which helps to nourish the body and make you feel good."

In terms of weight management, according to the *Journal of Alternative and Complementary Medicine* study, a whiff of the cool, refreshing scent of peppermint can ease mental exhaustion. This could strengthen your resolve to say no to that bowl of chocolates sitting on your co-worker's desk, or pass right by the pizza place you can't stop thinking about.

The drop in estrogen levels that are occurring during midlife can decrease your level of *serotonin.* This chemical in the brain is responsible for triggering fullness when eating and reducing cravings. Cravings are not really a question of mind over matter or willpower, which is what we've been led to believe. If your serotonin levels are naturally lower, there may be an actual biological reason for the cravings. We can stop blaming ourselves for "cheating" or for being "weak." On top of that, our moods change when estrogen levels drop, and we experience a lack of energy, which makes it even harder to resist temptation.

A drop of peppermint oil in my water, or applied directly to the roof of my mouth, helps me keep going, and I often find a few extra hours have passed without my even thinking about food. I used to chew gum or pop a mint in my mouth if I was hungry and couldn't eat immediately, but even the sugar-free versions can trigger insulin. That's why I switched to peppermint oil instead of gum and mints when I'm fasting and want to pop something in my mouth, but it is not time to eat.

Peppermint oil has been used for hundreds of years to support the digestive tract. An article from the *American Association of Family Physicians* discussed a study showing peppermint being "effective in relaxing intestinal smooth muscle by decreasing calcium influx into the muscle cells." When you first start IF and you're eating healthy, you may be trying foods that are new to your diet, including ones with more fiber. It's possible that this adjustment might cause some bloating and digestive discomfort. Peppermint oil can help support your digestive system. I rub it on my belly after a big meal all the time. Peppermint oil should probably be avoided if you have a hiatal hernia or significant GERD disease because its effects may exacerbate symptoms.

Peppermint is similar to the citrus oils in that it is excellent for cooking and flavoring water, but all of these oils can carry too strong a flavor into certain recipes. Refer to the end of this chapter for advice on the best ways to cook with oils.

Bergamot

Bergamot is best known for its use in perfumes due to its light orange and floral scent that mixes well with other scents. It is a citrus fruit and is what's used to flavor Earl Gray tea. It is the size of an orange but the color of a lime. Bergamot essential oil is perfect for the stress eater, those people whose stress triggers poor eating choices and who internalize their stress, creating the excess cortisol responsible for belly fat. Bergamot can work even better when paired with Lavender oil, as both oils help calm and relax the body and mind. According to Dr. Edwards of the Global Healing Center, the oil from the Bergamot plant has many uses, "including supporting balanced blood sugar, cholesterol and providing support to an individual's weight loss efforts." He continues, "High blood sugar is an indication that the body is retaining more glucose than it is eliminating, which in turn turns into stored fat." Research out of the University of Catanzaro in Italy (where the Bergamot plant originated) noted that after a month of using bergamot, subjects experienced reductions in LDL (bad cholesterol) and blood sugar levels, whereas HDL (good cholesterol) levels rose by over 40%.

Bergamot is so effective because of its high content of *polyphenols*, which are also found in green tea. Dr. Edwards says, "polyphenols are helpful compounds believed to halt production of blood fats, stimulate the metabolism, and prevent the absorption of cholesterol." Bergamot oil has an uplifting, lemon-lime scent and is delicious when added to water.

Bergamot is one of the essential oils that can calm you and give you peace of mind. This calming effect can help you to fend off overeating or eating to relax. It boosts weight loss efforts by easing emotional stress. Try a few drops in your water or in your diffuser or wear it as perfume.

Cinnamon Bark Oil

One whiff of cinnamon and I am transported back to my grandma's kitchen and us baking cookies together. Cinnamon Bark oil contains unique compounds not found in the dry spice version and is much more potent. Well-researched health benefits of cinnamon bark oil related to weight loss include a decrease in inflammation, reduction in blood sugar, and decreased LDL (bad cholesterol).

One of the leading causes of heart disease is obesity. Obesity is the product of inflammation and stress to the body. Insulin resistance (pre-diabetes) is a significant cause of obesity, and obesity is a major cause of insulin resistance. Interesting. . . . Hormonal changes are another cause of obesity. In a study found in the *Iranian Journal of Basic Medical Sciences* on the effects of cinnamon on metabolic syndrome (pre-diabetes), the authors concluded that "the anti-obesity effect of cinnamon was due to its insulin sensitivity, cardiovascular protection and immunomodulatory (immune response) effects."

One recent study found in the journal *Metabolism* suggests that "cinnamon can help fat cells burn energy because of the way that cinnamaldehyde, one of the compounds that give cinnamon its distinctive flavor, acts in the body."

Try a drop of cinnamon bark oil in tea or a smoothie. If it is too strong, try dipping a toothpick in the cinnamon oil and swirling it into the tea or hot water and add honey. Also, diffusing the oil before eating may help you eat less.

Ginger Oil

Ginger has a unique peppery sharp/sweet scent. In an article in *Time* Magazine, titled "How Ginger Fights Body Fat," the author cites a review in the *Annals of the New York*

Academy of Sciences which examined the effect ginger had in 60 different studies. They concluded that "overall these studies have built a consensus that ginger and its major constituents exert beneficial effects against obesity, diabetes, cardiovascular disease, and related disorders." The authors continue to describe that the ginger spice plays a role in fat burning, lowering cholesterol, and may even reduce the build-up of dangerous fat in the arteries.

Ginger oil is made up of about 90 percent sesquiterpenes (the constituent that erases the misinformation written on our DNA cells, leading to physical problems). A 2013 study in India found that ginger essential oil is packed with antioxidants. They also found it reduces inflammation and improves the digestive system so that more nutrients can be absorbed. This ultimately reduces the food cravings triggered by a lack of nutrients.

Replace the ginger in your recipes with ginger essential oil for an added health boost, and add a drop to your tea to support your digestive system.

THE IF & ESSENTIAL OILS COMBO

Now that you have learned that there is scientific evidence behind essential oils supporting your body as natural detoxifiers, fat burners, blood sugar balancers, mood elevators, and craving-curbers, do you better understand why essential oils and Intermittent Fasting are the perfect pairing?

These are just a few of the essential oils that may help boost your results, both during the fasting part of your day and when you eat. Essential oils have helped me and my clients to not only survive but thrive during our fasts. I recommend that you experiment with the oils and see how they affect your mood, hunger level, and overall weight loss progress. Each individual is different, and the way essential oils interact with our bodies affects everyone differently, just like with food.

During my fast, the only oils I typically ingest are lemon, peppermint, lime (which we didn't talk about but which works similarly to the other citrus oils), and a citrus blend that contains grapefruit, orange, lemon, tangerine, mandarin, and spearmint oils. During my eating window, I cook with a number of different citrus, herb, and spice essential oils.

COOKING WITH ESSENTIAL OILS

There are over 100 essential oils considered GRAS (Generally Regarded As Safe) by the FDA and are considered safe to ingest and cook with when labeled for internal use. Essential oils can replace the herbs, spices and citrus zest and juice in recipes, but you need to know a few things before using oils in your cooking. Essential oils aren't measured in teaspoons for cooking because they are so concentrated. There are approximately 60 drops of oil to a teaspoon. The good news is because of essential oils potency, you'll only need a drop or sometimes even less to accentuate the flavor. As a general rule, less is more when it comes to using essential oils in your food or drink.

I'll use lemon oil as a substitute for lemon juice in a recipe as an example.

1. If a recipe calls for one teaspoon of lemon juice, use 1 drop of oil to start, mix, taste, and add another drop if needed.

2. Don't drip your oils right into the food. Drip them onto a separate spoon. Rarely does just one drop come out of the bottle, and 2 drops could overpower your dish.

3. If a recipe calls for one tablespoon of lemon oil, start with 3-4 drops and add to taste.

4. Add 4-6 drops of oil to replace the zest of fresh fruit, and slowly add more if desired.

5. If a recipe calls for one teaspoon or less of a stronger flavored herb or spice such as oregano, basil, rosemary, thyme, sage, dill, black pepper, cinnamon bark, clove, ginger, nutmeg, or peppermint, then use the toothpick method. Dip a toothpick in the essential oil and then swirl it into the recipe to blend with the other ingredients. Don't put the toothpick back into the bottle. If you want to add more oil, use the other end or a new toothpick!

6. If using oils to flavor water, you MUST use glass, stainless steel, or ceramic, not plastic cups. The oils will pull the toxins from the plastic into the liquid. If you are putting oils into a smoothie, the oils will be more diluted and mixed in so it is OK in a plastic cup, but don't let it sit there for a long time and be sure to wash out the cup when finished.

7. Use organic ingredients when cooking. This may not always possible due to lack of access to organic foods where you live or the cost, but do so whenever possible. The oils are supporting a gentle detoxification of your body, so it makes no sense to add toxins back in. You can also use the lemon oil to wash the produce.

8. When heated, essential oils will lose their potency. That is why it is best to add oils at the end of a recipe after removing the dish from heat, or at the end of the boiling, baking or simmering process.

Cooking with essential oils is easy, fun, and convenient and gives your meals, salad dressings, desserts, drinks a flavor kick and an added health boost.

RECIPES

These are a few easy, healthy, house favorite recipes I make with essential oils.

GUACAMOLE: Mash 2 avocados. Add 2-3 drops of Lime oil. Add in a little bit of salsa (or not) and salt to taste.

BLACKBERRY-LIME WATERMELON: Combine cut up watermelon and whole blackberries in a bowl. In a separate bowl collect the juice of 2 limes. Add 3-4 drops of Lime oil to the juice and mix. Pour over the fruit and serve.

BASIC VINAIGRETTE DRESSING: Combine 3 tablespoons extra virgin olive oil, 1 tablespoon apple cider vinegar (or balsamic, rice, sherry, or other wine vinegar), 3 drops of Lemon essential oil, salt, and pepper to taste.

Chapter 5

The 16/8 Method of Intermittent Fasting: A Starting Place

By this point, I hope you understand why Intermittent Fasting works and how beneficial it is for the midlife woman. The second half of this book will focus on HOW you do Intermittent Fasting, specifically the 16/8 method. There are other methods of Intermittent Fasting, but I find the 16/8 to be the most natural way of losing weight and maintaining results for a lifetime. As I mentioned at the beginning of the book, the 16/8 method refers to an approach in which you don't eat any food for 16 hours of the day (fasting time), followed by a period when you can eat whatever you want, provided you do so during an 8-hour eating window (feasting time). I teach a "clean" fast, which means ingesting only water, black coffee, unflavored tea, and essential oils during the 16 hour fast (remember, you'll be asleep for much of the actual fasting time). For the best and quickest results, during the 8-hour eating window I recommend mostly choosing foods that are healthy, filling, and which satisfy your cravings. Allow yourself wine, dessert, and other indulgences less often. The 16/8 method is flexible to fit your schedule. You pick the 16 hours you fast each day based on what your day looks like. You can plan for success!

STRETCH THEN SAVOR

I began this book by saying that Intermittent Fasting isn't focused on what foods you eat, it's based on WHEN you eat food. When you follow an eating schedule, you can theoretically eat whatever you want. Gin Stephens' book *Delay Don't Deny* was what started it all for me. She shared the details of IF in simple terms, and the concept of "Delay Don't Deny" totally clicked for me as the perfect fit for my life. I tweaked her motto a bit to "Stretch Then Savor," which soon became a mantra in my head. It refers to stretching out the time between meals a few extra hours so you can really savor your food during your eating window. This concept helped me in two ways. One, it was easier to get through my fasting times. Two, focusing on foods I could savor led me to make good food choices. With only 8 hours to eat, I wanted to make sure the foods I ate were going to sustain me until the next meal and provide me with adequate nutrition and caloric intake. I also wanted to really enjoy my food choices, and not fill up on foods I could care less about. If I mindlessly munched garbage, I would no longer be hungry for the good stuff. The idea of savoring is a pleasant surprise for many of my clients when they start out with IF. Many people who said they thought fasting would be hard because they love to eat find that, because they have a limited eating window, they're more likely to make their meals count, choosing foods they truly enjoy. Of course, some choices they make are healthier than others, but they enjoy every morsel.

THE STARTING LINE

Here are some ideas to set you up for success:

1. *Mentally prepare yourself and commit to IF for at least 30 days*

2. *Take your initial weight* (I recommend weighing in no more than once a week)

3. *Take your measurements* (chest, waist, stomach, hips, upper arms, thighs, calves – re-measure once a month)

4. *Take "before pictures"* (from the front, back, both sides – take a photo every month, you'll be surprised by the changes, even if only a few pounds were lost)

5. *Go grocery shopping* (I will give you food recommendations further along in this chapter)

6. *Let your family, close friends, and people you eat with at work know what you are doing so they can support you*

7. *Start weaning yourself off the cream and sugar in your coffee if you are going to continue to drink coffee during the fasting times. This will make the transition easier.* (Only black coffee is allowed during the fast, but no worries, you can still enjoy your coffee with cream and sugar, just wait until it's feasting time.)

In working with many women over the years, I have found that for some, taking a "before" picture or learning of their starting weight derails them. Instead of becoming a motivating factor, it stops them from taking action or just makes them feel bad. If that's your fear, don't record weight, measurements, or take photos. Look for other ways to recognize you're moving in the direction you want, like how much better your clothes or rings fit.

Some people are probably better off keeping quiet to the people they interact with about their new journey, as people criticize what they don't understand. Misery is said to love company, and sometimes people try to hold you back so they won't feel left behind. Of course, that's their issue, not yours, but sometimes it's better to just stay quiet about IF until you are comfortable with how others may react. My husband knew when I started Intermittent Fasting, but I didn't tell too many other people at first. I didn't feel like explaining myself when I wasn't 100% sure if it was going to work. I wasn't confident that IF was all I was hoping it would be, and I didn't want other people's opinions countering my efforts.

CLEANSES & DETOXES

People ask me if they should do a detox or cleanse before starting IF. That's totally up to you. It is definitely not a requirement for success. In general, I recommend doing a detox or cleanse every six months. It resets the body and mind. It makes sense to do one before starting IF because it usually helps decrease cravings by reducing or eliminating sugar, carbs, and animal proteins. If you get rid of these cravings before starting IF, it will be easier to make healthier choices in your eating window once you begin. Most detoxes and cleanses also have you eliminate coffee. Many people experience headaches and mood issues when they give up coffee. Although you won't need to stop drinking coffee when you start IF, you will need to drink it black within your fasting period. If you'd prefer to not drink coffee without cream and sugar during the fasting part of the day, then a pre-fast detox could help ease the adjustment. If you give IF a try for 6-8 weeks and aren't getting the results you hoped for or are having trouble reducing the number of sugary snacks, pastas, and breads you consume during your window (this is recommended for the best IF results), then consider doing a detox or cleanse. If you would like a free copy of my *7 DAY SUGAR DETOX*, go to **bit.ly/MidlifeMojoSugarDetox**. It includes a list of what foods and liquids to eat and drink, what items to limit, and what to avoid consuming, along with sample meal recommendations and tips for success.

FIGURING OUT YOUR IF SCHEDULE

I truly believe that if more people just paid attention to the messages their bodies send them, they would naturally eat in a 16/8 rhythm. But most of us don't. Do you eat a piece of toast or a small yogurt or a piece of fruit in the morning just because you're trained to start your day with some food, not necessarily because you're actually hungry? Maybe it became a habit, and now it's routine.

Start to listen to your body in the morning, and don't eat if you're not hungry. If you eat in the morning automatically, not because you are actually experiencing hunger, you may not find the adjustment to the 16/8 eating schedule all that painful. If you are someone who lives for breakfast, or who gets up at 5 am for work and are ravenous by 9, waiting until the afternoon to open your eating window may not be for you. No worries. One of the great things about the 16/8 window is its flexibility. You can choose the hours you eat versus the hours you fast. Maybe you're someone who wants to open the eating window early in the day and close it earlier too. You can choose to eat breakfast and skip dinner instead! No big deal. It's not about what you call your meals. It's about 8 hours in which you eat during a 24-hour period. You get to choose the fasting/feasting schedule. Start eating at 9 am and end by 5 pm if you like or begin at 4 pm and eat until midnight. Eat what you want, what you enjoy, at whatever 8 hour window of time works best with your schedule. That sure doesn't sound like any "diet" I ever heard of!

Although schedules change, it is easy to figure out the eating window that works best for you and to make adjustments when necessary. For instance, I'm a night owl, up until midnight or later. I pretty much open my eating window around 2 pm every day and close it by 10 pm, then fast from 10 pm until 2 pm the next day. But one Tuesday a month I attend a business luncheon where I pay good money for the meal, which is served at noon. I'm not going to miss out on the good eats, so the night before I just make sure to close my window by 8 pm so that I can eat at 12 pm the next day and enjoy the luncheon. It's that simple. Then I revert back to my regular schedule.

Grab a pen. At the end of this chapter is a 24-hour clock. Draw out your eating window. A visual is helpful. Think about your routine:

- *What time do you typically eat dinner?*
- *What time do you go to sleep?*
- *What about mornings?*
- *Are you an early riser, at work before most people are awake and famished by 9 am?*
- *Do you have a shift job that has you eating at weird hours?*
- *Are you up late into the night like I am?*

Think about which two meals are ultimately the most important to you – breakfast/lunch or lunch/ dinner. In my house we eat dinner late, and since I stay up late, I would rather have a 10 pm evening snack than eat eggs and toast in the morning. By 10 pm, I'm good to shut down the kitchen for the night and begin my fast. From there, I count forward 16 hours and that sets my eating window to start at 2 pm. Now I have a schedule. 2 pm to 10 pm I eat, and from 10 pm to 2 pm I don't eat. It doesn't get easier than that.

Figure out your schedule right now. Knowing your typical IF cycle makes things easier. It becomes cut and dry. You start eating at this time, you stop at that time, and you choose how much and what to eat in between. Knowing your IF cycle helps you plan ahead for changes to the schedule, so you never need to feel like you are cheating, just adjusting as needed. Now that's serious eating freedom!!!

There are days when you are going to get an unexpected invitation out to eat, or something else happens that revolves around eating outside your window. Don't panic, and don't let your eating regimen hold you back from enjoying a meal and quality time with others. Just adjust your window. Or just call it a short fast day. Don't feel guilty if you don't make it to the 16-hour mark every day because of how the day unfolded. Let it go and start fresh tomorrow. One day does not unravel anything you've done.

WHAT YOU CAN HAVE DURING THE FAST

Everyone wants to know: What can I consume during the fast? Well, don't get too excited – it wouldn't be a fast if you were doing a lot of consuming.

During the fasting hours, you can have:

- *black coffee* (no creamer, no sugar, no artificial sweetener, no stevia)
- *green or black tea, unflavored*
- *herbal tea* (no fruity or sweetened tea)
- *plain water*
- *sparkling water*
- *freshly squeezed lemon or lime juice*
- *essential oils* (experiment for yourself, but I tend to stick to citrus and peppermint oils exclusively)

That's my list. Some people allow themselves other things during the fast, but I try to promote as clean a fast as possible. I personally just drink plain water during my fasts, adding the occasional essential oil if I feel I need some flavor or if I'm struggling to make it to the end of my fast or want to extend it a bit I will add Peppermint oil.

Black coffee and teas may provide added benefits to a fast. For some people, caffeine helps them with energy and focus if they're regular coffee drinkers. It might help lift your mood during the first weeks of IF. Coffee even has some appetite suppressant effects. Caffeinated beverages such as green tea or coffee cause the body to release more fatty acids from stored fat into the bloodstream, so they can be burned up as energy. Personally, I feel that the less coffee and tea and the more water you consume the better for proper hydration. But it's good to know it is OK to enjoy these beverages. (I know my coffee drinking people will be in a panic otherwise.)

Some people say you can squeeze a lemon or lime in your water. One fluid ounce of lemon (30.5g) only has 2g of carbs, and since you dilute it in water, some believe the juice won't affect the fat burning process. I've included them both on my list but I personally would rather not take the chance, so the decision to substitute a drop of lemon or lime-infused essential oil into my water was, for me, an easy choice.

FAQ'S ABOUT THE FAST

After working with clients and participating in many online Intermittent Fasting groups, common questions arise. Here are my responses.

Do I have to fast every day?

If you're doing the 16/8 method of Intermittent Fasting, daily consistency is key to getting and keeping your body in fat burning mode. Skipping a day here and there won't unravel all your hard work, but from my personal experience and what I have observed with my clients, a day of skipping can easily turn into a week or more if you let it. I prefer not to think of it as "skipping," but rather as shortening your window that day if something comes up, and then quickly getting back on schedule. There are other methods of Intermittent Fasting that don't require fasting every day, but they also restrict calories which is something I don't like to do because I enjoy eating so much. Although such a method is effective for fat burning, I feel that mentally it's more difficult because each day is something different and planning your schedule is more difficult. Your mind never develops a routine, which is foundational for long term success. Remember, Intermittent Fasting isn't something you do to lose weight – it is a lifestyle for permanent change.

Can I take my medications during the fast?

I'm not one to play around with one's health, and would never advise someone to do so. Definitely continue taking your meds. If your instructions are to take them with food, do your best to either adjust your schedule around taking your meds, or eat them with a small amount of fat, like an avocado.

Can I take supplements during the fast?

To me, this is the same as taking medications. Either adjust your fast or eat a small amount of fat with your supplements.

I'm feeling lightheaded during my fast. What should I do?

First, try adding a drop of peppermint oil to some water and drink it down. If that doesn't help, then break your fast early, eat something, and start your next fast accordingly. Listening to your body is a central theme in how I teach IF.

I get so hungry during my fast. What can I do?

Drink water. Sometimes we mistake thirst for hunger, water quenches our thirst. Peppermint oil is my go-to. I mentioned its benefits in helping us complete our fasts without thinking about food non-stop. Put a drop in water and drink down the entire glass.

Will brushing my teeth affect the fat burning stage?

Please, for the world's sake, brush your teeth. Most kinds of toothpaste don't have any calories, but most everyday toothpaste does have sugar alcohols in them, which may be enough to send a sweet signal to the brain and trigger insulin release. I brush my teeth with a natural toothpaste that uses essential oils, baking soda, xylitol, coconut oil, and stevia – and I use a minimal amount. Yes, there is a small chance that this could possibly stop the fat burning, but it's not being swallowed, and I use the bare minimum. It hasn't affected my results. Whatever type of toothpaste you use choose to use, natural or commercial, use as little as possible.

Can I chew sugarless gum or mints during the fast?

In the way I teach IF, the answer is no. Some research has shown that chewing gum or mints creates a sweet taste, which may trigger insulin. Some people also say the act of chewing makes them even hungrier. Try using a drop of peppermint oil directly on the roof of your mouth instead to take your mind off eating, and to freshen your breath.

Is it safe to fast for longer than 16 hours?

Yes, longer fasts are definitely safe. After some time on IF, you may find yourself naturally starting to fast for 18 to 20 hours without really thinking about it, as your body has adapted to fat burning and continues to provide you with energy. Also, if you find that after 4 or 6 weeks of 16/8 you're not getting results, you may want to increase the length of your fast, if not every day then at least a few days a week.

THE BEST WAY TO EAT DURING YOUR WINDOW

Time to eat! But first, let's cover the eating window guidelines. I'll start off by saying that you literally CAN eat ANYTHING you want. But just because you can doesn't mean you should. Common sense tells us that the healthier the foods we eat, the quicker the results we will see. I know that it's not easy to commit to losing weight, especially in midlife with all of its distractions. The main reason for losing weight at this point in our lives should be to live long, healthy, active lives, and that means making better food choices. Do we also want to look and feel good about ourselves when we look in the mirror? Of course, but for most women at midlife and older, losing weight should be about both vanity AND wellness.

You've got 8 hours in your eating window to do with as you like. For most people on IF, that consists of two main meals and maybe even two snacks. Some even fit in three main meals. For some, it is one snack and one large meal. The main thing is to EAT during your window, but to choose wisely. Quick carbs like sugary foods, starches, and bread get burned off first, leaving you hungry just a few hours later. To feel satisfied so that you're not ready to eat your arm off during a 16-hour fast, make sure you get well-rounded nutrition during your feasting time by choosing foods that take longer to digest so that they'll sustain you. I recommend focusing on eating more fats and proteins and fewer carbohydrates, but how much of each is dependent on knowing and listening to your body.

HEALTHY EATING THE 80/20 WAY

I have always subscribed to the 80/20 way of eating, which refers to eating healthy 80% of the time and indulging 20% of the time. I carried this philosophy into my IF journey. My personal IF eating plan focuses on eating lesser amounts of healthy carbs, moderate amounts of non-animal proteins (I am a vegetarian), and higher healthy fat intake daily. I incorporate essential oils into my cooking as much as possible.

From the categories of foods below, try to eat mostly from category #1 through category #4, 80% of the time, and eat from categories #5 and #6 the other 20%. Choose foods that are non-GMO, organic, hormone free, in season, and locally grown whenever possible. We've discussed the effects toxins have on a midlife woman's body. It only makes sense to eat as clean a diet as possible and to avoid exposing ourselves to chemicals through our food.

1.   **Healthy, higher fat foods** – Always have a ripe avocado on hand – they will be your new best friend. Also have in your cabinet extra virgin olive oil, coconut oil, nuts, and chia seeds. You can also include cheese and full-fat yogurts, but I recommend limiting dairy.

2.   **Healthy, higher protein foods** – Eat meat, poultry, fish, tofu, protein powders, quinoa (yes it's a carb, but a healthy one and a good source of protein, fat, and fiber for vegetarians), and eggs. I recommend limiting animal products. When you do eat them, make sure they are hormone free, grass fed, and organic if possible.

3.   **Vegetables** – Eat leafy greens like spinach and kale, or cruciferous vegetables such as broccoli, and cauliflower. Limit starchy vegetables like potatoes and corn.

4. **Fruits** – Whole fruits and berries are best. Berries are high in antioxidants and good for anti-aging. Don't overdo the fruit because of their high natural sugar content. Avoid dried fruit, fruit juices, and high carb fruits like bananas most of the time, saving them for indulgences.

5. **Healthy, complex carbohydrates** – Choose whole grains, quinoa, brown rice, beans, legumes, and oats.

6. **Junk food, simple carbohydrates** – Limit bread, pastries, sugary sweets, pasta, alcohol, fat-free and low-fat salad dressings.

*Avoid processed foods and artificial sweeteners – they are just bad for you.

We live in the real world, so I allow for junky foods 20% of the time, but I recommend to avoid making them a habit. Most people will still lose weight even if they consume these types of foods, but they are not good for us over the long haul, and the goal of the eating window is to fuel the body for success, vitality, and longevity. I'd prefer you get your carbs from filling foods on the healthy carb list than diving into a Milky Way bar.

Review this list, and try and choose foods you enjoy that are also high in fiber. An article put out by the Mayo Clinic said that fiber gives us a feeling of fullness. It can help fight constipation and assists the body with elimination. It may also lower blood sugar levels and promote weight loss. The article recommends 21 grams of daily fiber for women over age 51, and 25 grams if you are younger than 50. It recommends foods that fall into categories 1 through 5 in the list above. Some specific, healthy foods which are high in fiber include our friend the avocado –10 grams to a cup! Raspberries have 8 grams of fiber per cup, one artichoke equals 10.3 grams, and chia seeds deliver a whopping 10.6 grams per cup. Other high fiber foods include popcorn, beans, lentils, oats, and whole grains. Even dark chocolate contains 3.1 grams of fiber per ounce.

The foods you choose to eat, and when during your window you choose to eat them, can make the difference in successfully limiting insulin spikes and burning away the stored fat. The foods you choose also impact your hunger level during your fast. Simple carbohydrates are the first place the body turns to for energy, and it burns them up pretty quickly. If you are eating high carb sources like bread, pastas, and ice cream as your last foods before closing your window, there is a good chance that the following day you'll feel sluggish and hungry long before the 16-hour mark. There is also a chance you won't even get into the fat burning mode by the 16-hour mark, which is a waste of a good fast. I suggest that if you choose to eat these foods, eat them at the beginning of your eating window. That's also the best time to have cream and sugar in your coffee. Then focus on eating fats, proteins, and veggies during the second half of your feasting time. If you use this strategy, not only will you feel satisfied longer, but because these foods don't usually trigger insulin release, you will be giving your body a more extended opportunity to get in and stay in fat burning mode.

FAQ's ABOUT THE EATING WINDOW

What are the best foods to eat to break the fast?

There is no right way to break the fast. You can eat whatever you choose. I usually break my fast with something small to get over the hunger hump so that I don't let myself mindlessly gorge. I will eat a piece of avocado toast, a piece of fruit, or a little hummus and veggies. Then, a little while later, I'll have my first meal of the day. I find I eat less at my meals because I am not ravenous.

What are the best foods to eat to end the feasting window?

Again, there is no steadfast rule about what you eat, only when you eat it. That said, I choose to end my fast with foods that are higher in fat and protein. I find that on the days when I eat lots of carbs at the end of the window, I am much hungrier much earlier the following day. Experiment with different foods at the end of your window and observe how you feel the next day. That is the best way to figure out what foods sustain you best.

Is there a certain amount of calories I should be eating every day?

Remember, when you do the 16/8 method of Intermittent Fasting there is no calorie counting. Instead of focusing on the quantity you are consuming, focus on the quality of the foods. Make sure you eat to satisfaction during your window. One can overeat healthy foods just as easily as unhealthy foods, which will slow results. This is NOT a starvation diet. Chapter 6 will teach you how to gauge your hunger and satisfaction level and how to eat according to what your body needs. The number of calories ingested daily will be different for everyone and will fluctuate daily.

Can I have any kind of alcohol?

CAN you? Yes. SHOULD you? Well, you decide after hearing what I have to say. There are definitely mixed opinions on this. It will be up to you to experiment with IF and alcohol and determine if it affects your results.

I keep saying that the body turns to the carbs we eat to burn for energy first, then to the other foods. Well, that is not wholly accurate. When you consume alcohol, the body must deal with it FIRST, before processing foods and other non-alcoholic drinks. Only then does the body turn to your stored fat for energy. While it's busy with processing the alcohol, your body puts all weight loss and fat burning on hold. Alcohol also creates carb cravings and undermines our willpower because we tend to let our guard down when we have a couple drinks. However, if you do choose to drink, there are definitely better, low carb (not necessarily low calorie) choices. Here's a list of 4 low-carb alcoholic drinks:

- *Champagne or dry sparkling wine* – one glass contains about 1 gram of net carbs.
- *Dry wine* – red or white – one glass contains about 2 grams of net carbs.
- *Whiskey* – one drink contains 0 grams of carbs.
- *Dry Martini* – one cocktail contains 0 grams of carbs.

Can I have my cream and sugar now?

YES!! Enjoy!! But remember, that needs to get burned off first before burning stored fat, so (a) don't go crazy and (b) consume these earlier in your window.

How much protein, carbs, and fats should I be eating daily?

You're asking the wrong girl. I'm not a numbers person – I depend on my ability to listen to my body. I make sure to eat a low number of carbs each day, a moderate amount of protein, and a higher amount of fat (which can also come from the protein).

Isn't eating more fats bad for my heart?

No, that's another myth. It's the sugars that clog up the heart, not the fats you consume. The quality of the fat matters too. There is a big difference between consuming fat from ice cream and fat from an avocado. That being said, don't overdo it.

What are some vegetarian sources of proteins?

If you Google vegetarian protein charts, you will find that protein comes from many different sources, including animal products, dairy, vegetables, fruits, whole grains, nuts, and seeds. According to Rachel Meltzer Warren, MS, RDN, author of *The Smart Girl's Guide to Going Vegetarian*, the following are the best sources of protein:

Tofu – There are 10 grams of protein per 4 oz. serving of firm tofu – Tofu is a soy-based product, and there are differing opinions on women and soy as well as menopausal women and soy. I am not going to spend time on this topic, but I do highly recommend you research and decide for yourself whether tofu or other soy-based products are right for you.

Beans – There are 7 grams of protein per ½ cup serving of cooked black beans.

Greek Yogurt – Greek yogurt has 17 grams of protein per 6 oz. in the 2% version. If you decide to eat dairy products, I recommend that you buy the full-fat version, as low fat and fat-free versions typically substitute fat with sugar and artificial sweeteners. For Greek yogurt, buy plain and sweeten it yourself with fruit or raw honey.

Eggs – You receive 6 grams of protein per large egg.

Lentils – Lentils have 9 grams of protein per ½ cup.

Nuts and Nut Butters – Nuts and nut butters have 7 grams of protein per 2 Tbs. serving of peanut butter.

Tempeh – Tempeh has 21 grams of protein per 4 oz. This is also a soy-based product.

Quinoa – Quinoa has 8 grams of protein per 1 cup.

Vegetables - Many vegetables contain more proteins than people realize. A few protein-dense examples are spinach, asparagus, broccoli, cauliflower –all contain around 5 grams of protein per serving.

How much water should I be drinking per day?

A lot! Strive to drink half your weight in ounces to be exact. Here's an easy calculation to figure out how many cups (8 oz. per cup) of water you should be drinking daily: Take your current weight, divide that number by 2 and that is how many daily ounces you should be drinking. For example, a 160-pound woman divides 160 by 2, which comes to 80 oz. (10 cups) of water daily. Adding essential oils to your water is a natural way to add flavor, and they can be added both during the fasting and feasting times to help increase your water intake.

What is the "whoosh" effect?

Well, I couldn't believe it when it first happened for me. I hadn't been releasing weight for a few weeks, even though I was eating and fasting really clean. One night I just totally indulged on all types of junk. I woke up the next day assuming the scale had gone up, but I noticed instead that my stomach actually looked and felt tighter and the scale showed I actually went down. What?? That didn't make any sense to me until I learned about the whoosh effect that happens for some people when they're fasting.

There was a study performed during World War II called the Minnesota Starvation Study. Thirty-six volunteers went on a restrictive caloric diet for 6 months with periods of hard labor. The intent was to study the physiological and psychological effects of starvation to better treat returning prisoners of war. One interesting finding regarding weight was that initially there was weight loss, but then it steadied out, and ultimately became erratic. Seemingly out of the blue, 3 pounds or more would be gone overnight. Now, people can't burn fat that quickly. These scientists discovered that when stored fat is released from the cells, the cells didn't just collapse. Instead, they filled up and retained water to maintain the cells' shape. The body, after all these years, assumes more fat is on its way to be deposited, so the cells keep their shape while waiting for more fat to be stored. After consistently doing Intermittent Fasting for some time, the body gives up and realizes that no fat is on its way. It collapses and releases the water that it was using as a placeholder.

When you do IF for a while, you may notice that the area where your fat used to be now takes on a sort of squishy consistency. Squishy fat forms because, as I described above, as the fat is being released, the cells are filling with water. You may feel softer than usual. Sometimes squishy fat forms in places we can see it, and sometimes it forms more internally where we can't. The squishy fatty areas can last from a few days to as long as a few weeks. And then one day you wake up and WHOOSH! You look and feel leaner!

Some people don't believe the whoosh effect is real, but most people who have been long-time dieters over the years have probably experienced unexplained, significant, weight drops when trying to lose weight. Some dieters believe a large "cheat" meal can trigger this phenomenon.

Not everyone experiences the whoosh effect, and I don't recommend sabotaging your healthy eating habits and purposefully trying to create this effect. I'd instead strive for consistency. Just eat healthy 80% or more of the time, stick with the 16/8 fasting schedule, and you will see results.

GRADUAL BUILD-UP

Not everyone feels comfortable diving right into 16 hours of fasting, and that's OK. (Though I assure you, you won't starve to death!) It's okay to "ease into" the IF lifestyle. If 16 hours seems like too long for you, my suggestion for midlife women beginning IF is to aim for a 12- to 14-hour fasting window for the first week or so. I realize many people will just dive right into 16-hour fasts and do fine, but it is good to give your body and mind an adjustment period to this totally new thing you are starting.

See how your body handles the change during the first week. Are you struggling in the last few hours of the fasting window? Are you feeling woozy? Are you hangry? Doing OK? Then gradually increase your fasting period to 16 hours a couple days during the next week. Still good? Then continue doing the 16-hour fast and increase to 7 days a week. As you get more comfortable with IF and your body settles into its new routine, you can start to extend your fasts beyond 16 as long as your body is OK with it. I generally don't recommend midlife women fasting for more than 24 hours, but I have clients who do well with extended fasts. It's just not my thing.

We've now covered the ins and outs of an Intermittent Fasting lifestyle. Use the following 24-hour clock to help you figure out your starting IF schedule. The next chapter will teach you how to make Intermittent Fasting a permanent part of your life.

CREATE YOUR IDEAL DAY. MARK OFF YOUR HOURS OF FASTING AND YOUR EATING WINDOW. Remember, this isn't set in stone, but it should correlate to your usual and most likely schedule.

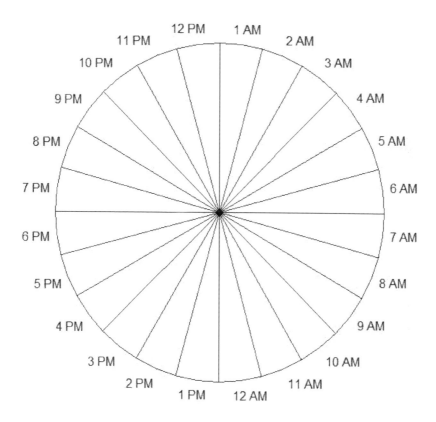

Chapter 6

Get Off The Diet Train Forever!

I told you at the beginning of this book that I was going to help you get off the diet train forever. This next chapter will guide you to making Intermittent Fasting a permanent lifestyle.

I keep saying to listen to your body and pay attention to what it's telling you. But how do you actually DO that? I suggest purchasing a notebook to start tracking your foods and exercise and to journal your physical experiences and emotions as you begin Intermittent Fasting. Using your notes as a guide, you will be able to shape your IF journey and make changes along the way to find what foods and exercise make you feel good and give you the results you want. You'll be able to figure out how long your body needs to fast to lose fat and feel great. There is no cookie cutter approach to creating an Intermittent Fasting lifestyle because everyone's IF journey and lifestyle looks different. You need to invest the small amount of time and effort it takes to track and journal the first few months of doing IF for the big payoff down the road when you not only lose the stubborn midlife middle, but lose it forever.

SATISFACTION SCALE

The Hunger Scale

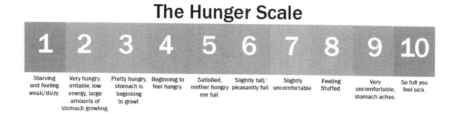

1	2	3	4	5	6	7	8	9	10
Starving and feeling weak/dizzy.	Very hungry, irritable, low energy, large amounts of stomach growling.	Pretty hungry, stomach is beginning to growl.	Beginning to feel hungry.	Satisfied, niether hungry nor full.	Slightly full/ pleasantly full.	Slightly uncomfortable.	Feeling Stuffed.	Very uncomfortable, stomach aches.	So full you feel sick.

One tool to help you get in tune with your body's true needs is the Hunger Satisfaction Scale. It will help you to extend your fasts, eat in moderation, and feel good AFTER eating.

When it's time to break the fast during your first few weeks of IF, you are going to feel like going hog wild – don't. Use the following satisfaction scale to keep you from gorging and feeling sick. Use it to create a new pattern of eating that becomes second nature.

It's simple: When your 16 hours of fasting are up, rate how you are feeling on a scale of 1 to 10 before you eat. A rating of 1 means you're so hungry you can't think or speak, and if someone put a bowl full of crickets in front of you, you'd gobble them down. A rating of 10 means you feel you feel stuffed and sick to your stomach. You ideally want to start eating when you are feeling a 3 (slightly hungry), which after a 16-hour fast is how most of us feel.

Start eating. Halfway through your meal stop for a moment and rate yourself. Are you a rating of 5/6 and perfectly satisfied? If so, stop eating, put the fork down, and do the dishes. Both your body and mind are satisfied. Are you still hungry?? If so, eat a bit more until you reach a 5 rating, feel full but still good. Have you eaten past satisfied and are feeling like an 8, 9 or 10? A rating of 10 has you feeling so full you need to unbuckle your pants, and they have to carry you away from the table. Learn from that awful feeling, and next time check in with yourself sooner.

Give yourself a final rating when you're finished eating and again one hour later. Do you feel sluggish? Are you energized? Are you experiencing any digestive issues? Taking a rating one hour after eating will help steer you towards choosing foods that make you feel great and avoiding ones that make you feel poorly.

The best time to stop eating is when you feel good and the hunger twinges have subsided. However, most of us instead put our forks down, pause for a moment, but we don't walk away. We let the food sit there, tempting us. Oh, and we remember how Mom told us there are starving children somewhere in the world and that we shouldn't waste food. Out of habit, we mindlessly pick up the fork again and chow down until we reach last few bites and then . . . Oops! We've passed satisfied and are suddenly deep into fully bloated, nausea territory.

Keeping track will initially help you utilize your eating window to its fullest, and you'll feel great.

FAST LENGTH TRACKING

There are different ways you can track your fast lengths. There are apps (see the *Resources* chapter), premade charts and graphs you can download, or you can write in your journal, noting the time you stop and start your fast each day. If you don't track your fasts, it can become hard to recall. It's nice to have at a glance a record of whether you did more 14-hour days than 16-hour days, or if you hit your 16 every day, or perhaps did longer fasts on a few days, so you can see how the different times affect your results.

FOOD AND WATER TRACKING

I'm not going to ask you to write down every little bite, lick, and taste you have, although you may choose to do so. But I do suggest that in your journal you keep a general list of the foods you eat, snack on, and the liquids you consume during the eating window at the beginning of your IF experience. Again, this allows you to eyeball your results and assess whether you've eaten a good balance of fats, carbs, and protein during the day and if you drank enough water. You don't need to write down the minute details, just the foods in general. For example, if you have for lunch a salad with greens, beans, avocado, and chicken, write that down. You don't have to write every veggie in the salad unless you want to. Also, write down how you physically feel 60 minutes after the meal. Did your food choices energize you, make you feel sleepy, or hurt your stomach? Is there a pattern of certain foods that cause you to either feel great our lousy an hour later? Tracking means information gathering so you can review your eating and determine what, if any, changes are needed. Make sure to include any alcohol you drink and the time it was consumed (i.e., the beginning, middle, or end of your feasting window), especially if it's a higher carb drink like beer. Remember, it is usually going to take you longer to get to burning the stored fat when you consume alcohol.

EXERCISE TRACKING

I'll address exercise more in the next chapter, but it's a good idea to note in your journal your daily physical exertions. Those could include playing a sport, doing Pilates, going to the gym, dancing, or working for hours in the garden or doing heavy housework. Also, note how long you engaged in the activity. The more you record, the more information you'll have to work with. If one week you did at least 30 minutes of activity every day and had great results, and the next week you lost nothing and saw you only worked out twice, you can pinpoint the possible cause and adjust your schedule instead of feeling like a failure, or that IF doesn't work and giving up.

TRACKING FEELINGS

We have addressed the mental and physical impact of stress on weight loss and how emotions can lead to poor choices and overeating. Keeping track of how you feel throughout the day can give you more insight into your IF results. It can also help you recognize areas of your life you may want to address using a different response other than turning to food. Did you feel overwhelmed at work, so you went to the vending machine? Were you pissed off at your spouse, so you drank a bottle of wine? Or did sadness over the recent loss of a pet cause you to find solace in a bag of Oreos? Depressed about your body size? Proud of an achievement? Excited about a new opportunity? Any feeling on which you spent time and mental energy during the day is one you should write down: the good, the bad, and the ugly.

RESULTS TO EXPECT

So, what kind of positive changes should you expect with IF, and how quickly? First of all, know that nothing happens overnight. IF isn't a magic pill or magic wand. It isn't a fad or a lose-weight-quick gimmick. Intermittent Fasting results in real, permanent weight loss, and it takes patience and persistence (notice that I didn't say "perfection") to achieve it. It took years to pack on your unwanted pounds, so losing them safely, at a reasonable rate of ½ to 2 pounds a week, takes time. You may initially see a big drop, and then things won't change much, followed by another drop. Or you may be like me, the turtle, the slow and steady weight loser. If you have a lot more to lose, you may see the weight drop faster than someone trying to lose the last 10 pounds. Who cares how it happens, really, as long as you get to where you want to be?

Everyone's results will be different. It depends on your current health level, how much you have to lose, how clean you fast, how clean you feast, the stress levels you're dealing with, the environmental toxins you are exposed to, the personal care and cleaning products you use, the hormonal issues you have going on, the medications you are on, and your own unique genetic makeup.

In the 28-day Jumpstart program I teach, called *Melt The Midlife Middle,* I've had clients who lost close to 20 pounds in 4 weeks, ones who lost 8, and ones who lost none but then, 9 weeks in, they caught up and the weight and inches began to fall off. Just stick with it and I promise you will lose the unwanted pounds.

Having taken your initial measurements, you will be able to gauge your losses in both pounds and inches easily. Those are the visible results. There will also be lots of non-scale/non-ruler victories too, some which are even better than seeing the numbers change. Here are just a few of the great outcomes that could lie ahead on your IF journey:

- Feeling more in control
- More energy
- Clearer thinking
- Increased confidence
- Your clothes and jewelry get looser
- Your skin is clear and glowing
- Less muscle and joint pain
- Reduced need for medications
- Less frequent heartburn
- You are more fun to be around

- Fewer mood swings
- Discovering new foods you love
- Less snoring
- Saving money on groceries and eating out
- Buying new clothes

WHAT IF YOU'RE NOT LOSING WEIGHT?

You read this book and possibly go on to some of these IF support pages on Facebook, where you see people sharing amazing results, but then you give it a try and nothing happens. The scale doesn't budge. What can you do to get things moving?

First, be honest with yourself. Are you really 100% all-in and committed and sticking to the 16/8 IF plan? If the answer is Yes, then look at these potential adjustments to get the results you want:

- Extend your daily fast to 18 hours
- Do an extra-long fast (20+ hours) 1-2 times a week
- Look back through your journal and tweak your food choices
- Make sure you aren't overeating within your window
- Have nothing but water during your fasting time. No coffee, no tea, just plain, pure water
- Cut back on alcohol or, even better, eliminate it completely
- Make sure you are tracking your foods, exercise, and fast length
- Increase your exercise
- Make sure your expectations are realistic (5 to 8 lbs. a month is considered a healthy and safe rate of weight loss)
- Get accountability by joining my *Melt The Midlife Middle* support group
- Get your hormone levels tested

- Make a doctor's appointment to see whether there may be an underlying medical issue
- Give it time, at least 8-12 weeks

MAINTENANCE

I teach IF as a permanent lifestyle. But what happens when you reach your goal weight, and no longer want to lose any more? How do you maintain your weight while continuing to receive the benefits of autophagy, as well as the non-scale benefits such as the mental clarity one feels when living the IF lifestyle?

Don't worry, you don't have to stop fasting, you just need to do some tweaking. You need to find your balance between the number of hours fasted and the amount of food you eat during your window. I have found maintenance to be easy. My body is accustomed to using fat for fuel, so all I need to do is shorten my window a few days a week to 12-14 hours instead of my usual 16-18 hours. I also indulge a little more often, with my food choices or in the quantity I eat, than I did when my goal was primarily to lose weight. If I see the scale go up, I'll tighten up the IF reigns until I'm back on track. It all traces back to listening to your body and observing how changes, fast length, and food choices affect your body. I will NEVER go back to the traditional way of eating 3 meals and snacks again!

COMMUNITY SUPPORT

Support is vital to your success, but you must choose wisely when it comes to where you get yours. Most people don't understand what IF is, so it's not unusual for them to assume you are starving yourself and to try to dissuade you. Some people will intentionally (or unintentionally) derail you from your efforts, for example, by baking your favorite treats, so you'll feel obligated to eat them. Some people will comment on your choices, making you feel uncomfortable when you meet for breakfast and all you drink is coffee. Surrounding yourself with a community of people who are all doing IF can make the transition easier. I discuss more about finding your IF community in Chapter 9.

Whatever you do, stick with it. Even if you never lose a pound, the anti-aging and health benefits alone are well worth it. But you WILL lose weight – just be patient with your body, and keep reassessing and making changes.

YOU GOT THIS!!

CHAPTER 7

A Few Things To Consider

SAFETY FIRST

When most people first hear about fasting, they equate it with starvation and therefore conclude it's not safe. I know that's what I thought before I did my due diligence. Let me be clear: *Intermittent Fasting is a perfectly safe way to lose weight when done correctly,* but it's not for everyone. I don't recommend IF for individuals in the following categories:

- *You're pregnant* (probably not a problem for the midlife woman)
- *You have a history of eating disorders*
- *You are chronically stressed and/or have adrenal issues*

Some people will experience mild side effects as their body adjusts during the first week or so to its new IF routine. When starting IF, I suggest a gradual build-up in the length of your fasting window. Some side effects/annoyances you may experience include:

- *Feeling weak*
- *Headaches*

- *Feeling "foggy" mentally*
- *Mild fatigue or irritability*
- *Flu-like symptoms*

Thankfully, these types of side effects are temporary and are alleviated quickly as your body adapts to the dietary changes. Believe me, you will survive and it will be worth it!

The midlife woman has to pay extra attention to her body. Every person's genetic makeup is different, the foods they eat are different, their toxic environmental exposure is different, their stress levels are different, etc. Therefore, everyone's IF experience will be different. Most women enjoy great success once they commit to the IF lifestyle.

Midlife women have an extra element to consider when they first experiment with IF. All of our hormones are interconnected, and our diets and eating patterns can affect these connections. When we're already experiencing anxiety, sleepless nights, and sweat pouring down our backs all day due to our out-of-whack hormones, the last thing we want to do is exacerbate it all. This is why learning to listen to your body is so important.

In the beginning, I dove right into 16-hour fasts. My night sweats definitely worsened. Clients of mine have jumped right in with 16-hour fasts with no issues at all. If I were to do it over again, I would gradually build up the length of the fasting window over the first couple of weeks. It doesn't hurt to go slow, and that's what I recommend doing. Experiment a bit with your fasting window to see if IF reduces your menopause symptoms or exacerbates them. If it heightens your symptoms significantly, consider a more gradual approach. Pay close attention to how your body is responding to intermittent fasting. Watch for any of these changes:

- Increased stress

- Trouble falling or staying asleep
- Hair loss
- Anxiety or depression
- Low energy
- Slowed digestion
- Muscle pain or increased soreness
- Mood swings
- Loss of sex drive
- Loss of menstrual cycle (although it can be challenging at this age to determine what is normal and not)
- Feeling cold

If you are experiencing one or more of these symptoms in a pronounced way after trying IF for a few weeks, you should immediately make some adjustments, either to the length of your fasts or the foods you're eating.

PHYSICAL ISSUES TRACKING

I just listed the possible negative signs to watch out for, some of them specific to the midlife woman. Write down in your journal any negative issues you are currently experiencing, physical and emotional, and rate the issue (i.e., hot flashes, trouble sleeping, anxiety) prior to beginning IF on a scale from 1-10 (a rating of 10 means the issue is very bad and interferes significantly with your daily functioning). You should check in once a week and rate yourself again. Are you feeling better and the numbers are going down? Are some issues getting worse? Have others disappeared completely? Wouldn't it be great if your acne cleared up or your migraines disappeared as an added bonus to losing your midlife middle?

Intermittent Fasting is a completely safe and effective way for the midlife woman to lose weight. This chapter isn't meant to scare you off or give you an excuse not to try IF, but to make you aware of things to look for so you can tweak your fasts and/or feasts and feel great when doing IF. Pay attention to what your body is saying, and it will tell you what it needs.

Chapter 8

The Clock Is Ticking, It's
Time To Get Moving!

You can no longer afford to be a couch potato when you hit 40. It's time to make exercise a priority. Exercise is vital not only for losing weight, but for your overall physical and mental well-being, so get out there and move your body!

Getting your heart rate up, strengthening muscles, stretching, practicing balance, and doing physical activities you enjoy are ways to make exercise a part of your daily life. Exercise will help you attain the fit body you desire and may also prevent future surgeries or falls. I recommend moving your body in some way every day, even if it's simply taking the stairs instead of the elevator, or choosing to park your car a bit further from the entrance to the grocery store. I suggest more formal exercise 4-5 times a week. Even light exercise is good for the midlife woman's heart, bones, stress level and mood.

We discussed the many benefits exercise has when combined with IF in general, and specifically for the midlife woman. Some of the benefits are:

- Exercising in a fasted state burns more stored fat
- Exercise increases insulin sensitivity

- Your athletic performance improves when you exercise while fasting
- Exercise increases the production of Human Growth Hormone
- Increased lean muscle mass results in burning more calories

BEST TYPE OF EXERCISE FOR MIDLIFE WOMEN

The middle-aged female body has different needs than that of men and younger women. General strength training has been shown to increase HGH levels in both men and women. Remember, fasting also raises HGH levels, which builds muscle mass, boosts metabolism, burns fat. This increase in HGH levels created by fasting helps slow down some of the visible signs of the aging process. However, women need more intense strength training to raise their growth hormone levels.

To create a release of HGH, you must first increase your body temperature. You need to get moving and kick things into high gear, go beyond your comfort zone, and get out of breath. Exercise in short 10-30 second bursts of 90% to 100% maximum intensity effort. This might look like 30 seconds of jumping jacks or push-ups, followed by a 15-second rest, repeated for 2 to 4 minutes. This cycle allows your body to experience a phenomenon called "oxygen debt." It is this oxygen debt that triggers the HGH release.

HIGH-INTENSITY INTERVAL TRAINING

High-Intensity Interval Training (HIIT) is an excellent workout for the midlife woman to create that oxygen debt and raise those HGH levels. HIIT is known to burn fat in a short time. These workouts significantly boost one's metabolism, allowing the body to keep burning fat even after the workout is completed. HIIT workouts get your heart beating, improving cardiovascular health and endurance.

I want to connect some dots here. Earlier, we talked about why exercising in a fasted state is so effective. Research shows that 20% more fat is burned when exercising on an empty stomach. If you couple that with the fat burning that occurs during a HIIT workout, you get a double whammy of fat burning. And because a HIIT workout doesn't take up much time, it can be a very effective way to improve your overall success and ability to maintain long-term results. Both fasting and exercise increase fat burning and create the conditions for the release of HGH and its anti-aging effects. Are you ready to pull on those leggings and tank top and get your body moving?

HIIT workouts help you reach that 90-100% maximum effort level through short bursts of effort, followed by periods of rest to keep it manageable. You may not be able to run on the treadmill for 60 minutes straight, but I bet you can muster up the energy to spend 10 minutes giving it all you've got.

Here is an example of an 8 minute HIIT workout:

20 seconds jumping jacks

10 seconds rest

20 seconds squats

10 seconds rest

20 seconds jog in place with high knees

10 seconds rest

20 seconds pushups

10 seconds rest

Repeat 4 times.

HIIT is great for fat burning and so much more, but we need to balance this high-intensity workout with workouts that focus on lean muscle building, flexibility, balance, and mental relaxation.

STRONG BONES

One of the reasons exercise is so important is that it helps women maintain good bone health. The article "The Assessment of Fracture Risk" from the *Journal of Bone and Joint Surgery* claims that osteoporosis "affects up to 40% of postmenopausal women." I mentioned earlier that a study done in 2016 revealed a possible link between periods of fasting and improved bone health. Studies done in 2003 and 2011 showed that "certain types of exercise might result in improved bone strength even after menopause, a time when bone mass declines and the ability to rescue lost bone is impaired." So once again, the combination of exercise and IF proves useful for the midlife woman's overall health. The best exercises for building bones and keeping them strong, according to the National Osteoporosis Foundation, are high impact, weight-bearing and muscle strengthening exercises. It is essential to know your body. If you have had hip, knee, or foot surgeries, or if you already have moderate to severe osteoporosis or a heart condition, you may need to avoid high impact exercises. However, low impact, weight-bearing exercises can also help keep bones strong and are a safe alternative if you're unable to do high impact exercises safely.

SAFE & EFFECTIVE EXERCISES

High Impact Exercises

- *Dancing*

- *High Impact Aerobics* (lots of jumping and feet leaving the ground)
- *Jogging/Running*
- *Jumping Rope*
- *Tennis*

Low Impact Exercises

- *Elliptical Machine*
- *Low Impact Aerobics* (no jumping)
- *Stair Step Machines*
- *Fast Walking on a Treadmill or Outdoors*

Muscle Strengthening Exercises
(Resistance Exercises)

- *Lifting Weights – I recommend lighter weights* (2-5 pound hand weights) *and more repetitions and sets rather than lifting heavy weights*
- *Using Elastic Exercise Bands*
- *Using Weight Machines*
- *Body Weight Exercises* – planks, lunges

Mind-Body Exercises

We have learned how excess stress to the body and mind slow down our fasting progress. We also know that as we age, our posture worsens, and so does our balance and flexibility. The following exercises help to improve posture, balance, flexibility, and assist in de-stressing and calming the mind. Consider diffusing calming or uplifting essential oils, like Bergamot, when doing these exercises.

- *Pilates*
- *Yoga*
- *Tai Chi*

I suggest a weekly workout that has an adequate balance of:

- *Stretching before and after workouts*
- *Intense, high energy HIIT workouts*
- *Strength training*
- *Mind/Body workouts*

If you haven't exercised in a while – or EVER – start slowly. Perhaps first consult your doctor. Going at it full force from the get-go isn't a great idea. You'll most likely hurt yourself or get discouraged. Do it right. Build up your strength, build up your endurance so you can eventually do full cardio/strength training workouts. Expect some soreness if you are new to exercising. If getting to a gym is difficult for you and working out with a video at home alone isn't motivating, then check out my two-way, live, interactive online Pilates mat classes. Links to more information are in the *Resources* chapter.

Essential oils can also help support you during and after your workout. Peppermint oil can be inhaled or ingested in water to energize you for your workout. Essential oils that support your respiratory system, such as eucalyptus oil mixed into coconut oil can be rubbed on your chest to support endurance when doing cardio exercises. Wintergreen oil, known for supporting healthy muscles and joints, can be mixed with coconut oil and rubbed on your body after a tough workout.

The foods you consume during your eating window affect both your workout and your post-workout recovery. It is important to eat a balance of quality protein, complex carbs, healthy fats, vegetables, and fruits during the eating window to maintain a healthy fast. On the days you work out, make sure to increase your healthy, complex carb intake (more beans, quinoa, etc. . .) for greater sustenance and satisfaction. On the days you don't exercise, choose more protein, vegetables, and fats and fewer carbs.

Working out regularly builds not only strength and endurance – it also increases one's confidence and feelings of empowerment and being in control. Intermittent Fasting and exercise can be the one-two punch for finally losing the midlife middle.

Chapter 9

Shed The Emotional Weight

So what do IF and emotions have to do with each other? For many women, body perception, emotional health, and self-worth are deeply intertwined. As mentioned earlier, these connections may date back as far as childhood or the teen years. Do you have emotions that are intertwined with weight issues? I'm betting most of us do. Were you ever bullied for being overweight? Did a parent, knowingly or unknowingly, make you feel not good enough because you weren't "model skinny?" Maybe a stranger made an unkind comment at a time when you were feeling vulnerable. I can remember being a teen and comparing my curves and extra padding to my best friend who could eat anything and remain super slim. I chose to wear long, flowy, hippie skirts and ponchos under the guise of being "comfortable," but I wasn't happy with my body and purposefully "hid" myself. I see pictures of me at that age now and realize that I too was thin, but at the time I felt overweight and self-conscious. I saw that best friend for the first time in many years a few months before starting IF. She was still slim, while I had extra pounds on me. Old insecurities I thought I'd put to rest resurfaced. So many of our interactions over the years find their way into our subconscious, and they dictate the thoughts we have about ourselves and the paths we take.

Have you ever called yourself fat? Have you ever let your weight stop you from taking a chance on a relationship? Have you ever feared you would die because your weight made you feel so unhealthy? Have you, have you, have you? I've seen so many examples of how women connect their bodies, thoughts, decisions, and actions. Frankly, it makes me sad.

I have a close friend who is 25 years older than I am. She once told me that in midlife, all the crap you've been pushing down comes up and forces you to deal with it. She also said that midlife is a freeing time because you start to care less about what other people think and you stop trying to please everyone. I don't know about you, but as I get older I realize that you can never please everyone –the best thing you can do is find your own peace and happiness.

What thoughts are coming up for you as you read this book and contemplate starting your own Intermittent Fasting journal? Are you thinking, "this can work for other people but not for me?" Are you worried that your spouse will give you a hard time if you tell him/her you are fasting? Are you assuming that you don't have the willpower?

If you haven't delved into the emotional side of your weight gain or inability to lose the weight, now is the time. Holding down your emotions leaves you feeling stuffed. I am a massive fan of professor, author, and public speaker Brene Brown. This quote by her says it all:

"I think midlife is when the universe gently places her hand upon your shoulders, pulls you close, and whispers in your ear: I'm not screwing around. It's time. All this pretending and performing these coping mechanisms that you've developed to protect yourself from feeling inadequate and getting hurt – has to go. Your armor is preventing you from growing into your gifts. I understand that you believed your armor could help you secure all of the things you needed to feel worthy of love and belonging, but you're still searching,

and you're more lost than ever. Time is growing short. There are unexplored adventures ahead of you. You can't live the rest of your life worried about what other people will think. You were born worthy of love and belonging. Courage and daring are coursing through you. You were made to live and love with your whole heart. It's time to show up and be seen."

Powerful! Brene talks about "your armor." For many midlife women, that armor can be the extra pounds she carries to "protect" herself. Or the excuse she makes to not go out and meet new people, or to avoid starting a new relationship. I love the final line: "Show up and be seen." Allow that to really sink in. Now is the time to heal your body and mind from the inside out. None of us can count on tomorrow. Be the best version of yourself today. The truth is that weight is only an arbitrary number on the scale that can change day to day, even hour to hour. Feeling well and enjoying life should be your priorities. You shouldn't let your well-being be dictated by the metal box on the bathroom floor. Being your best self looks different on everyone. I say live healthfully AND happily ever after!

I am not a therapist, but I strongly suggest you speak with one if you feel there's significant trauma in your past that needs a trained professional's guidance, or even if you just feel that you need some extra emotional support. It's important to manage the emotional side of your IF journey. Look deeper within yourself so IF doesn't become just another diet that you start and stop.

"Food for the body is not enough. There must be food for the soul." – Dorothy Day, American journalist

WAYS TO NATURALLY MANAGE & RELEASE EMOTIONS

Essential Oils – As much as I love using oils to support my body, I tend to use them even more for boosting my emotional well-being. Our DNA stores memories and emotions. When you inhale an essential oil, it takes approximately 22 seconds to process and affect the emotional center (limbic system) of the brain. That's less than a minute before you can change the mood you're in or veer away from the negative thoughts and feelings you're having. That could be the difference between sticking to your fast or saying screw it, and breaking your fast early. The limbic system is directly connected to the parts of the brain that control heart rate, blood pressure, breathing, memory, stress levels, and hormone balance. Board certified pharmacotherapy specialist Dr. Lindsey Elmore says, "Because of this unique direct relationship between emotions and olfaction (sense of smell) within the brain, essential oils can help 'unlock' stored memories and emotions."

This explains why smells often conjure memories or feelings and why aromatherapy can have, in addition to its physiological advantages, such profound psychological benefits. Have you ever smelled a cologne that reminded you of an old boyfriend, or caught a whiff of something in the air that whisked you back in time to your family's beach house where you spent every summer? That's the power that scents exert on the brain.

Because high-quality essential oils are so concentrated, potent, and easy to use, they can provide a quick path to managing our feelings. There's a wonderful book that can help called *Releasing Emotional Patterns with Essential Oils*. Author Carolyn Mein, DC, recommends the appropriate oil to use for specific emotional issues, where on your body to put them, and even includes a positive affirmation statement to say aloud to help reprogram negative belief patterns. I highly recommend it for supporting your IF journey.

You don't need a specialist to use oils – just open up a bottle and sniff, or put a few drops into a diffuser. There are so many great options to choose from. I spoke of Bergamot oil helping with stress management. It is naturally uplifting and can also help one regain feelings of self-love, self-acceptance, and self-worth so that they feel confident and empowered. You can also purchase diffuser jewelry to wear, which I absolutely love. You just add a drop of oil to a diffuser bracelet or necklace and enjoy it all day long.

You can visit with an aromatherapist for more guidance, or look up Aroma Freedom Technique (AFT) Certified practitioners. These are specialists who pair certain oils with a specific protocol for releasing emotions and creating new, positive emotional pathways.

Affirmations – Our beliefs are merely repeated thought patterns we've reinforced since childhood. Some serve us, some limit us. A disconnect can occur between what we want and what we feel we deserve. Positive affirmations, combined with essential oils, can be powerful tools for spiritual and personal growth to help close the disconnection. Positive affirmations are statements of truth which one aspires to absorb into their life. They aren't just a wish upon a star. According to self-help expert Louise Hay, "An affirmation opens the door. It's a beginning point on a path to change." Affirmations are a way of tell your subconscious, "I'm ready." Coupled with the appropriate essential oil, affirmations are best said aloud, and even better spoken in front of a mirror so that you are genuinely facing yourself. Create your own affirmations or look up ones to use online.

A few sample affirmations include:

- *I love and accept myself exactly as I am.*
- *I am capable of achieving anything I set my mind to.*
- *I can be, do, and have anything I desire.*

Journaling – Writing is a powerful tool. Do you remember keeping a diary when you were younger? You wrote down all the thoughts and feelings you had but didn't want anyone to know. It felt good to get them out of your brain and out onto paper. Pennebaker and Beall's (1986) study demonstrated that expressive writing about a stressful experience improves indicators of physical health. If you have emotional healing to do, I suggest buying a journal and carving out daily time for free-flowing thought release, not on the computer but using good old pen and paper. While writing, make sure there's an essential oil in the diffuser. Don't analyze where your thoughts and feeling are coming from, just let them go and write. If you need help getting started, there are numerous journaling prompts you can find on the internet to help.

Here are a few examples:

- *When was a time you felt really proud of yourself?*
- *What advice would you give to yourself at 13 years old?*
- *What did you learn about food and eating from your mother?*

Find a supportive community – Motivational speaker Jim Rohn claims that "You are the average of the five people you spend the most time with." If that's true (and based on my experience, it is), make sure you choose your people wisely. When you embark on a new journey, it's essential to have people supporting you and cheering you on. It's hard enough to keep our eye on the IF prize day in and day out amidst all the temptations, stressors, and distractions so avoid negative people. Avoid people who say "you can't." We don't need to add to the challenges of changing and improving ourselves while dealing with the negative emotions thrown at us at home, in the office, or while we're simply living our daily lives.

Also, Intermittent Fasting, although the concept has been around for some time, has recently received a lot of attention, so there's lots of information and misinformation coming out daily. Most people around you are going to think you're crazy when you mention fasting, and they'll tell you it's not safe. If you listen to them, you may create doubt in your mind about whether IF is right for you.

You need first to find the people who understand *how* and *why* Intermittent Fasting works and who can explain it to you clearly because there's so much info out there. Second, you need accountability and the support of others who have had success with IF, as well as those still transitioning to an IF lifestyle. Finding a community is a crucial predictor of success. Many of us carry around so much baggage, and when we share that with others, we find that we are not alone in our struggles. A dedicated community can help you get past the make-or-break point when you're having a rough time in your fast. A community becomes your emotional cheerleader when you're down, and it can motivate you off the couch to get to the gym when you'd typically find an excuse not to go. A community exists to tell you that tomorrow will be a better day when you're being hard on yourself for breaking your fast early one day and will hold you accountable to get back on the path you want to be on the next day. IF is easier, more fun, and more effective in the long term when you connect with a community of like-minded people working toward the same goal. When we feel emotionally supported, we tend to make better choices. We get by with a little help from our friends!

My *Melt the Midlife Middle* private Facebook community includes women from ages 40-80, all trying to improve their physical and emotional well-being with IF. It is only for those who are currently going through or have completed my 28-day program. It's a place for long-term, continued support for members who intend to continue their journey long past the initial 28 days. Having a group of people who not only share practical info but who also give you the emotional support you need is golden. Check out the *Resources* chapter later in this book to get involved.

Letting go of the emotional weight you've been carrying for years can be the catalyst that motivates you to get physically healthy and fit once and for all.

It's Not The Ending, It's Only The Beginning

Intermittent Fasting can be life changing if you give it a chance. You have nothing to lose but pounds. The 16/8 method of IF as I teach it isn't brain surgery. There are 4 simple rules:

1. Don't eat for 16 hours.

2. Eat during an 8 hour period, choosing healthy foods 80% of the time and indulging 20% of the time.

3. Use essential oils to support your efforts during the fast and the eating window.

4. Listen to your body and adjust your fasting schedule and the foods you eat accordingly.

That's it! No counting, weighing, or measuring – just eat and don't eat. It doesn't get easier than that. The midlife woman already has enough on her plate to deal with between hormonal changes, managing her home and family, succeeding in her career, taking care of aging parents, etc. Eating shouldn't be a physical or emotional chore or burden. IF saves you money and time with fewer trips to the grocery store and less effort in the kitchen. It gives you more freedom to focus on the important people in your life and to do the activities you love.

Get off the diet train once and for all and lose the belly fat for good! Commit today to 30 days of Intermittent Fasting and see the IF magic unfold as you experience true eating freedom. You will soon be asking yourself where IF has been your whole life. All that matters is that you've found it.

The Top 100 Frequently Asked Questions About Doing the 16/8 Method of Intermittent Fasting & Incorporating Essential Oils for Losing the Midlife Middle for Good

INTRODUCTION

Are there different ways to do Intermittent Fasting?

What is the 16/8 method of Intermittent Fasting?

What are the major components of the way you teach the 16/8 method of Intermittent Fasting?

Where can I get more information on menopause?

CHAPTER 1

Is Intermittent Fasting another new, fad diet?

What does a typical day in the life of an Intermittent Faster look like?

Are there any foods I can't eat when doing Intermittent Fasting?

Is Intermittent Fasting hard to do?

Will Intermittent Fasting help me lose the last 5-10 pounds?

Will Intermittent Fasting work if you have 100 or more pounds to lose?

CHAPTER 2

How does our body process the foods we eat?

Won't my metabolism slow down if I don't eat every few hours?

Isn't breakfast the most important meal of the day?

Why does eating 3 meals and 2-3 snacks a day prevent us from burning stored fat?

How does Intermittent Fasting affect my blood sugar levels?

How will I survive 16 hours without eating? Won't I feel "hangry?"

Why doesn't the eat less/move more method work well for most people?

Will I lose muscle mass if I start Intermittent Fasting?

Will I burn more fat if I exercise on an empty stomach?

If I exercise in the morning, will I have enough energy to sustain me if my stomach is empty?

Can I do "hard" exercise such as distance running or body building while in a fasted state without feeling lightheaded?

If I don't eat right after exercising, will I still be able to focus and concentrate?

Should there be any difference in how you fast or feast on workout days vs. non- workout days?

CHAPTER 3

Why has it been so difficult to lose weight since I entered my 40's?

How does menopause affect a woman's weight?

How do toxins from the environment and personal care and cleaning products affect the midlife woman's weight?

What is autophagy and why is it important for the midlife woman's body?

What is the Human Growth Hormone and how does it benefit the midlife woman?

Will Intermittent Fasting help me to look younger?

My libido has been lacking since entering midlife. How can Intermittent Fasting help?

How does stress affect the midlife woman's ability to manage her weight?

Can Intermittent Fasting help with bone health for the midlife woman?

What exercises are most beneficial for the midlife woman?

What are some non-weight related benefits to adopting an Intermittent Fasting lifestyle?

CHAPTER 4

What essential oils are most effective for weight management for the midlife woman?

What is the science behind why essential oils are effective for getting rid of toxins and putting our body in balance?

How do you use essential oils in general?

I see essential oils for purchase in stores all the time. Are all essential oils created equal?

Will ingesting essential oils break my fast?

How can essential oils be used in Intermittent Fasting?

Are there any guidelines for cooking with essential oils?

What can I do to support my digestive system as I increase my consumption of high fiber foods?

How can essential oils support the emotional side of my weight loss journey?

Are there any easy recipe suggestions for using essential oils during my eating window?

CHAPTER 5

What should I do to prepare for Intermittent Fasting?

Should I do a detox or cleanse prior to beginning Intermittent Fasting?

Should I start with a 16-hour fast or work my way up to it?

Do I have to skip breakfast to do Intermittent Fasting?

What foods or drinks can I consume during the fasting period?

Can I take my medications during the fasting period?

Can I take supplements during the fasting period?

What should I do if I feel light-headed during my fast?

I get so hungry during my fast – what can I do?

Will brushing my teeth affect my getting into the fat burning stage?

Will drinking lemon water break my fast?

What foods are best to consume during the feast?

Can I drink alcohol?

Can I eat sweets?

Can I have cream and sugar in my coffee?

Can I chew gum or eat mints during the fast?

Are there any foods I can't eat during my eating window?

How much water should I be drinking each day?

How much protein, fats, or carbs should I be eating daily?

How much fiber should the midlife woman consume daily?

What are some examples of vegetarian protein?

Should I be eating organic foods?

Can I eat fruit during my eating window?

What is the best way to break the fast?

What foods are best to consume just before closing your eating window?

Are there a certain number of calories I should be eating daily?

Will eating foods with higher fat content affect my heart?

What is the "whoosh" effect?

CHAPTER 6

Do I need to keep a food diary?

How can listening to your body help you be successful at Intermittent Fasting?

Are there any apps that can track my fast length?

What kind of weight loss can I expect?

What are some things I can do if I find I'm not losing weight through Intermittent Fasting?

Should I be tracking my exercise?

I am an emotional eater. How can I change this?

What non-weight related benefits are there to Intermittent Fasting?

Is there a maintenance program for Intermittent Fasting once you achieve your weight goal?

Are there any Intermittent Fasting communities for support?

CHAPTER 7

Is it safe to fast for longer than 16 hours?

Will there be any side effects when I start Intermittent Fasting?

Is there anyone who shouldn't do Intermittent Fasting?

How will I know when I begin Intermittent Fasting if the physical issues I am currently experiencing will get worse or better?

CHAPTER 8

Is it safe to exercise when fasting?

What exercises are best for the midlife woman?

Will I lose muscle mass if I start Intermittent Fasting?

How often should I be exercising?

Should there be any difference between how you fast or feast on workout days vs. non-workout days?

CHAPTER 9

What are some ways I can shift my mindset about food and my relationship with eating?

What does Intermittent Fasting have to do with improving my emotional state?

How can essential oils support my emotions?

What are affirmations and how can they help me be successful with Intermittent Fasting?

How important is community support to my Intermittent Fasting success?

Do you suggest keeping a journal of my emotional journey while doing Intermittent Fasting?

CONCLUSION

What are your general rules for Intermittent Fasting success?

RESOURCES

How can I find online support when starting Intermittent Fasting?

Are there any apps that can track my fast length?

What other books/videos do you suggest?

Where can I purchase a high quality essential oil?

Do you offer any online Intermittent Fasting programs for beginners?

Do you offer any online exercise programs?

Where can I get more general support for my midlife years?

HAPPY "MELT THE MIDLIFE MIDDLE 28 DAY JUMPSTART PROGRAM" CLIENTS

"OMG . . . I am 139 pounds!!! I never thought I'd see "13-anything" ever again! 21 pounds in less than 3 months! What!! I went shopping and I bought some size 8's. It's been at least 15 years!" – Hillary M.

"It's been 2 weeks, I've lost 7 pounds and I really believe I can have control over my weight on IF." – Janelle W.

"Thanks to Jill and this awesome group, I feel like I am organically making small lifestyle changes that will actually stick!" – Amy S.

"I like that it is simple. I like the structure of eat/fast/eat, etc." – Janice M.

"I got on the scale today expecting weight gain, but I went on vacation and lost weight (2 pounds)!! This is the first time I have EVER done this! I overindulged several times but I extended my fasts and I lost weight on vacation. This is HUGE for me! So grateful to have discovered IF" – Marty E.

"Stepped on the scale this morning and I have released 6 pounds!!! Thanks for creating this program and support group of like-minded women!! It makes me feel good to know I am on this journey with so many wonderful women from all over the country and the world." – Faith J.

"With 2 months of IF under my belt, I am a believer. I have lost just about 8.5 pounds and despite weekends, vacations, Saturday nights out, etc., I am holding steady. People have told me they can tell I've lost weight. This is going to be a long haul for me, but I feel like for the first time in a long time I am seeing results and don't feel deprived." – Jocelyn D.

"I love the Peppermint oil. It really helps me not be hungry and get through my fast." – Melissa J.

"The citrus oils have given me hope that I can drink enough water. Staying hydrated is a challenge for me." – Agnes H.

"Tomorrow is 3 months since I started this new way of life. I have never been more happy or in control. Down 25 pounds since starting IF. I move my window around every day depending on what's going on and who is home. I have long windows and short windows. I can't imagine ever going back to three meals a day. I just love it!" – Jennifer F.

Resources

FASTING APPS

Zero

VORA

LIFE

Window

BOOKS (available on Amazon)

The Obesity Code: Unlocking The Secrets Of Weight Loss by Dr. Jason Fung

The Complete Guide To Fasting: Heal Your Body Through Intermittent, Alternate Day and Extended Fasting by Dr. Jason Fung & Jimmy Moore

Delay Don't Deny: Living An Intermittent Lifestyle by Gin Stephens

No Sweat! It's Just Menopause: Eating, Exercise & Essential Oils For A Healthy Change by Jill Lebofsky

Releasing Emotional Patterns With Essential Oils Carolyn Mein, DC

ONLINE VIDEOS

Dr. Eric Berg YouTube Videos

ONLINE PROGRAMS

Melt The Midlife Middle 28 Day Jumpstart Program – **bit.ly/ IFMeltMidlifeMiddle**

Midlife Mojo Virtual Pilates - **bit.ly/MidlifeMojoVirtualPilates**

ESSENTIAL OILS

Young Living Essential Oils – **bit.ly/YLJillLebofsky**

Bibliography

Bergamot. Retrieved July 19, 2018, from https://www.fragrantica.com/notes/Bergamot-75.html

Berg, E. (2018, March 22). Can I Drink Alcohol on Keto (Ketogenic Diet)? Retrieved from https://www.youtube.com/watch?v=jnZk-meNYcE&t=3s

Berg, E. How Long Does It Take to Get Into Ketosis [INFOGRAPHIC]. Retrieved from https://www.drberg.com/blog/how-long-does-it-take-to-get-into-ketosis

Berg, E. How Long to Get Into Ketosis After Your Cheat Day. Retrieved from https://www.drberg.com/blog/how-long-to-get-into-ketosis-after-your-cheat-day

Berg, E. (2018, August 19). What Is Glycogen? Retrieved from https://youtu.be/B4eO1SM09g0

Brown, B. (2019, May 24). The Midlife Unraveling. Retrieved from https://brenebrown.com/articles/2018/05/24/the-midlife-unraveling/

Champ, C. (2016). *Misguided Medicine.*

CFR - Code of Federal Regulations Title 21. Retrieved from https://www.accessdata.fda.gov/scripts/cdrh/cfdocs/cfcfr/CFRSearch.cfm?fr=182.20

Eenfeldt, A. (2018, December 30). Low-Carb Alcohol – Visual Guide to the Best and the Worst

Drinks – Diet Doctor. Retrieved from https://www.dietdoctor.com/low-carb/alcohol

Elmore, L. (2019, February 21). Emotions and Essential Oils. Retrieved from https://lindseyelmore.com/emotions-and-essential-oils/

Estrogen | Hormone Health Network. Retrieved from https://www.hormone.org/hormones-and-health/hormones/estrogen

Faubion, S. S. (2016). *The Menopause Solution*. Rochester, MN: Mayo.

Fujioka, K., Greenway, F., Sheard, J., & Ying, Y. (2006). The effects of grapefruit on weight and insulin resistance: Relationship to the metabolic syndrome. Retrieved from https://www.ncbi.nlm.nih.gov/pubmed/16579728/

Fukuchi, Y., Hiramitsu, M., Okada, M., Hayashi, S., Nabeno, Y., Osawa, T., & Naito, M. (2008, November). Lemon Polyphenols Suppress Diet-induced Obesity by Up-Regulation of mRNA Levels of the Enzymes Involved in beta-Oxidation in Mouse White Adipose Tissue. Retrieved from https://www.ncbi.nlm.nih.gov/pmc/articles/PMC2581754/

Fung, J. (2018, April 25). The Biggest Loser Diet - Eat Less Move More's Bigger Badass Brother - Fasting 22. Retrieved from https://idmprogram.com/the-biggest-loser-diet-fasting22/

Fung, J. (2018, November 16). The Biology of Starvation Calories Part V. Retrieved from https://idmprogram.com/the-biology-of-starvation-calories-part-v/

Gomez, J. (1970, April 03). New Research Finds Routine Periodic Fasting is Good for Your Health and Your Heart | Intermountain Healthcare. Retrieved from https://intermountainhealthcare.org/

news/2011/04/new-research-finds-routine-periodic-fasting-is-good-for-your-health-and-your-heart/

Grapefruit and weight loss. (2004, January 24). Retrieved from https://www.medicalnewstoday.com/releases/5495.php

Hay, L. The Power of Affirmations. (2017, August 23). Retrieved from https://www.louisehay.com/the-power-of-affirmations/

Intermittent Fasting (Time-Restricted Eating). Retrieved from https://burnfatnotsugar.com/assets/if.pdf

Intermountain Medical Center. (2011, May 20). Routine periodic fasting is good for your health, and your heart, study suggests. Retrieved from https://www.sciencedaily.com/releases/2011/04/110403090259.htm

Jackson, S. E., Kirschbaum, C., & Steptoe, A. (2017). Hair cortisol and adiposity in a population-based sample of 2,527 men and women aged 54 to 87 years. *Obesity, 25*(3), 539-544. doi:10.1002/oby.21733

Johnson, T. C. (Ed.). (2019, February 15). Causes of Menopause Weight Gain & Exercise Benefits. Retrieved from https://www.webmd.com/menopause/guide/menopause-weight-gain-and-exercise-tips#2

Levine, B., & Klionsky, D. J. (2017, January 10). Autophagy wins the 2016 Nobel Prize in Physiology or Medicine: Breakthroughs in baker's yeast fuel advances in biomedical research. Retrieved from https://www.ncbi.nlm.nih.gov/pmc/articles/PMC5240711/

Mawer, R. (2018, September 11). 11 Ways to Boost Human Growth Hormone (HGH) Naturally. Retrieved from https://www.healthline.com/nutrition/11-ways-to-increase-hgh

Mayyasi, A. (2016, May 9). How Breakfast Became a Thing. Retrieved from https://priceonomics.com/how-breakfast-became-a-thing/

Mein, C. (2017). *Releasing Emotional Patterns with Essential Oils.*

Mollazadeh, H., & Hosseinzadeh, H. (2016, December). Cinnamon effects on metabolic syndrome: A review based on its mechanisms. Retrieved from https://www.ncbi.nlm.nih.gov/pmc/articles/PMC5220230/

Nair, P. M., & Khawale, P. G. (2016). Role of therapeutic fasting in women's health: An overview. Retrieved from https://www.ncbi.nlm.nih.gov/pmc/articles/PMC4960941/

Osteoporosis Exercise for Strong Bones. Retrieved from https://www.nof.org/patients/fracturesfall-prevention/exercisesafe-movement/osteoporosis-exercise-for-strong-bones/

Pennebaker, J. W., & Beall, S. K. (1986). Confronting a traumatic event: Toward an understanding of inhibition and disease. *Journal of Abnormal Psychology, 95*(3), 274-281. doi:10.1037//0021-843x.95.3.274

Polidoulis, I., Beyene, J., & Cheung, A. M. (2011). The effect of exercise on pQCT parameters of bone structure and strength in postmenopausal women—a systematic review and meta-analysis of randomized controlled trials. *Osteoporosis International, 23*(1), 39-51. doi:10.1007/s00198-011-1734-7

Quotes by Dorothy Day. Retrieved from http://www.famousquotes123.com/dorothy-day-quotes.html

Raman, R. (2017, September 24). Why Your Metabolism Slows Down With Age. Retrieved from https://www.healthline.com/nutrition/metabolism-and-age

Rawlings, A. (2006). Cellulite and its treatment. *International Journal Of Cosmetic Science, 28*(3).

Rohn, J. Quotation. Retrieved from https://www.goodreads.com/quotes/1798-you-are-the-average-of-the-five-people-you-spend

Sanfilippo, Diane. Home of the Balanced Bites Podcast. (2018, December 12). Retrieved from https:// balancedbites.com/category/health-wellness/keto/

Santos, L., Elliott-Sale, K. J., & Sale, C. (2017). Exercise and bone health across the lifespan. Retrieved from https://www.ncbi. nlm.nih.gov/pmc/articles/PMC5684300/

Schofield, G., & G. H. (2016). "Understanding glucagon (and somastatin 28). *The Science of Human Potential.*

Sorvino, C. (2017, May 18). Why the $445 Billion Beauty Industry Is A Gold Mine For Self-Made Women. *Forbes.*

The Weight Loss Benefits of Bergamot Essential Oil. (2015, December 04). Retrieved from https:// www.globalhealingcenter.com/natural-health/ weight-loss-benefits-bergamot-essential-oil/

University of Michigan. (2017, November 21). Cinnamon turns up the heat on fat cells. Retrieved from https://www.sciencedaily.com/ releases/2017/11/171121095145.htm

Unnanuntana, A., Gladnick, B. P., Donnelly, E., & Lane, J. M. (2010, March). The assessment of fracture risk. Retrieved from https://www.ncbi. nlm.nih.gov/pmc/articles/PMC2827823/

Uusi-Rasi, K., Kannus, P., Cheng, S., Sievänen, H., Pasanen, M., Heinonen, A., . . . Vuori, I. (2003). Effect of alendronate and exercise on bone and physical performance of postmenopausal women: A randomized controlled trial. *Bone,33*(1), 132-143. doi:10.1016/s8756-3282(03)00082-6

Vegetarian Times Editors. (2015, March 12). 7 Top Protein Sources for Vegetarians. Retrieved from https://www.vegetariantimes.com/health-and-nutrition/7-top-protein-sources-for-vegetarians

Volant, L., Sanfilippo, D., Jenn, Sanfilippo, D., Dena, Sanfilippo, D., . . . Sanfilippo, D. (2018, December 12). Beautycounter | Diane Sanfilippo. Retrieved from https://balancedbites.com/beautycounter/

Wang, J., Ke, W., Bao, R., Hu, X., & Chen, F. (2017). Beneficial effects of ginger Zingiber officinale Roscoe on obesity and metabolic syndrome: A review. *Annals of the New York Academy of Sciences,1398*(1).

Warren, R. M. (2014). *The Smart Girl's Guide to Going Vegetarian: How to Look Great, Feel Fabulous, and Be a Better You.*

Berg, E. (Director). (2018). *What Is Glucagon?*[Video file]. Retrieved from https://www.youtube.com/watch?v=QQTUqyarPdY

Whittel, N. (2018). *Glow15: A Science Based Plan to Lose Weight, Revitalize Your Skin and Invigorate Your Life.*

Women and Heart Disease. Retrieved from https://www.cdc.gov/heartdisease/women.htm

Connect With Me

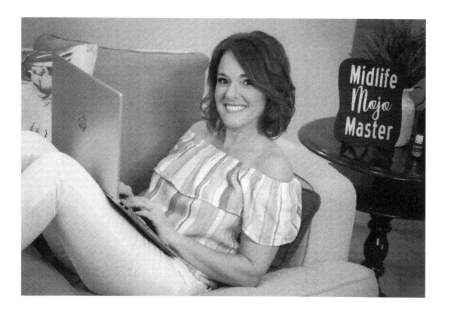

Sign up for my mailing list at bit.ly/
TheIFSecretSauce and receive a free PDF:

"The 5 Key Ingredients in The Secret Sauce for Finally
Losing the Stubborn Midlife Middle For Good"

Jill is available to speak at your
next online or live event!

Website

www.jilllebofsky.com

Email

jill.lebofsky@yahoo.com

Facebook

The Right Side of 45: (Private Group for the Midlife Woman) **bit.ly/rightsideof45**

Healthy U (Business Page) – **www.facebook.com/uhealthyu**

Instagram

The Right Side of 45: **bit.ly/TheRightSideOf45instagram**

Pinterest

The Right Side of 45: **bit.ly/TheRightSideOf45pinterest**

LinkedIn

Jill Lebofsky: **bit.ly/JillLebofskylinkedin**

YouTube

Midlife Mojo: **bit.ly/TheRightSideOf45youtube**

NO SWEAT!
IT'S JUST MENOPAUSE

EATING, EXERCISE AND ESSENTIAL OILS FOR A HEALTHY CHANGE

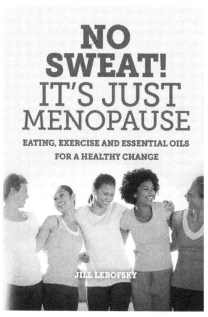

JILL LEBOFSKY

Jill's first book in her Midlife Mojo Series is available in print or e-book at **bit.ly/naturalmenopausebook.**

Jill is available to speak at your next online or live event.

HOT FLASHES. LOW LIBIDO. MOOD SWINGS. EXPANDING WAISTLINE. HELP!

For years, pre- and post-menopausal women have suffered in silence.

It doesn't have to be that way!!

When a woman's body functions optimally, menopausal symptoms should not be an issue. When your body is in balance, the years leading up to and following menopause should be the best years of your life.

No Sweat! It's Just Menopause takes a fun and simple approach to natural, plant-based solutions for some of the greatest challenges women face during this transition. Menopause doesn't have to mean the beginning of the end. Author Jill Lebofsky has successfully guided hundreds of clients through the menopausal years, revitalizing marriages, rebuilding confidence and enhancing physical and emotional wellbeing.

You will learn:

- A quick, easy fix for the #1 contributor to most menopausal symptoms
- Practical plant-based solutions to restore optimal hormonal balance
- How to incorporate essential oils into your everyday routine to support a healthy menopause
- The most effective foods and exercises for getting rid of the menopausal "spare tire"
- Healthy, natural ways to reduce hot flashes and night sweats
- Ways to increase libido and vaginal lubrication to return to a great sex life
- How to get fluctuating moods under control and feel empowered in your life

Don't run in a hot, sweaty panic to the doctor's office. Traditional solutions may help, but they often cause other, unwanted, problems. Try these natural suggestions as your FIRST stop on your road to a peaceful, invigorating, problem free menopause.

Made in the USA
San Bernardino, CA
12 February 2020